MW00947913

Arm Yourself for Fit & Faithful Living

How God-Seeking Women Should Equip Themselves for True Health

Sarah Hansel

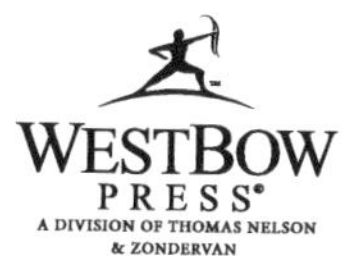

WestBow Press books may be ordered through booksellers or by contacting:

WestBow Press
A Division of Thomas Nelson & Zondervan
1663 Liberty Drive
Bloomington, IN 47403
www.westbowpress.com
1 (866) 928-1240

ISBN: 978-1-5127-6939-5 (sc)
ISBN: 978-1-5127-6938-8 (e)

Library of Congress Control Number: 2016921359

Print information available on the last page.

WestBow Press rev. date: 03/22/2017

TABLE OF CONTENTS

PROGRAM SETUP AND PRE-EVALUATION xiii

SECTION ONE: THE WAR ON YOUR HEALTH 1

Week 1–Preparing for Battle 4

Day 1: Accepting the Spiritual War 5

Day 2: Summoning Sooner 8

Day 3: Scraping off the Wallpaper 11

Day 4: Courageous Commitment 14

Week 2–Arm Yourself with Physical Health 18

Day 1: Fitness Organization 19

Day 2: Discipline Yourself 22

Day 3: Goldilocks 26

Day 4: The Comparison Scale 30

SECTION TWO: BELT OF TRUTH 36

2-Week Nutrition Challenge 37

Week 3–Arm Yourself with Truth 38

Day 1: Truth of the Gospel 39

Day 2: Blenders of Truth 41

Day 3: Don't Take the Bait 44

Day 4: Who's Leading Whom? 47

Week 4–Arm Yourself with Nutritional Health 52

Day 1: Banking on Your Health 53

Day 2: The Master Nutritionist 56

Day 3: Truth Behind Your Calories 59

Day 4: What To Eat? 62

SECTION THREE: BREASTPLATE OF RIGHTEOUSNESS 68

2-Week Emotional Challenge 69

Week 5–Arm Yourself with Righteousness 70

Day 1: Righteousness 71

Day 2: Detox of the Heart 74

Day 3: Organizing Your Desires 77

Day 4: Commanded or Compelled? 80

Week 6–Arm Yourself with Emotional Health 84

Day 1: Emotional Wars 85

Day 2: Emotional Jealousy 88

Day 3: Emotional Addictions 91

Day 4: Emotional Remembrances 93

SECTION FOUR: GOSPEL OF PEACE 98
2-Week Relationship Challenge 99
Week 7–Arm Yourself with Peace 100
Day 1: Gospel of Peace 101
Day 2: Running Wildly 104
Day 3: Actions are Louder than Megaphones 107
Day 4: A Time to Share 109
Week 8–Arm Yourself with Social Health 114
Day 1: Faith Friends 115
Day 2: Flourishing or Floundering Friendships 118
Day 3: Muzzle Thy Mouth 121
Day 4: Giving the Best in Each Relationship 124

SECTION FIVE: SHIELD OF FAITH 130
2-Week Stepping out in Faith Challenge 131
Week 9–Arm Yourself with Faith 132
Day 1: Shield of Faith 133
Day 2: The Crossing Spirit World 136
Day 3: Divine Communication 140
Day 4: Be Refreshed and Filled 142
Week 10–Arm Yourself with Spiritual Health 148
Day 1: The Idol 149
Day 2: Race of a Life Time 152
Day 3: What are You Multiplying? 155
Day 4: Discipleship 157

SECTION SIX: HELMET OF SALVATION 162
2-Week Mentally Strong Challenge 163
Week 11–Arm Yourself with Salvation 164
Day 1: Helmet of Salvation 165
Day 2: Organization of the Soul 168
Day 3: Immortal Entitlement 171
Day 4: Time Investments 174
Week 12–Arm Yourself with Mental Health 178
Day 1: Character Counts 179
Day 2: Conquering Mental Assaults 182
Day 3: Serving up Some Stew 185
Day 4: Performance Treadmill 188

SECTION SEVEN: SWORD OF THE SPIRIT 196
2-Week Full Armor Challenge 197
Week 13–Being Fully Equipped 198
Day 1: Sword of the Spirit 199
Day 2: Truth Alters Your Thinking 202
Day 3: Righteousness Helps You Become Emotionally Fit 205

Week 14–Arm Yourself with Whole Health 208
Day 1: Peaceful People Are Social Heroes 209
Day 2: With Faith Your Spiritual Health is Alive 212
Day 3: Salvation Makes You Mentally Savvy 214

TREASURE CHEST 222

ACKNOWLEDGMENTS 324

ABOUT THE AUTHOR 326

ENDNOTES 328

Hello, Beautiful Friends!

As a freshman in college, I distinctly heard the first whisper in my heart to write a book for women. It was not just a single whisper, however; it was an often impression on my heart that would come and go. Writing may sound simple enough for some, but I had a problem, or should I say, I *was* the problem. According to my high school English teacher, I could not spell, had no idea how to organize my thoughts, and my mind was too busy to accomplish much of anything important relating to writing. She told me to leave the advanced class because she was not sure how I got in any way, and go to a more simple class where they would help me—she did not have the energy. I tried to suppress my feelings of inadequacy, but her words lingered. This is where a battle between my heart and mind began.

"It's time," would be whispered more frequently as I finished up college and began life with my husband. *But I'm not author material.* I prayed for direction and clarity on this call because I was sure I could not do it without spell-check and divine intervention. *Why me?* I could not escape the call one evening as God led me to Ephesians 6 during my Bible reading time—the famous Armor of God passage. It was as if God spoke to my very soul. I based my writing to women and their health on this Scripture.

I have read of the Armor of God in Scripture many times before and even had most of it memorized. I remember learning the Sunday school stories when I was young and seeing mysterious clingy felt figures of Roman soldiers on the green board. *Where is the special link with health and telling women to dress up in imaginary armor? It seems too manly, and besides, it's an overused passage in the church world.* However, these Scriptures never left my thoughts.

I searched, prayed, and earnestly studied this passage until one night, as I sat in bed, it hit my spirit like electricity. I was so excited and inspired by how these verses linked the Armor of God and our health that I could not sleep. It ended up changing my entire perspective on fitness and became the purpose for this book. The basis of my book was not to be regular Bible study material or a fitness-focused wellness book; I was to combine both these avenues.

Teaching and coaching in the fitness and health industry, I have found that women are stuck and in need of freedom from more than just body fat. They need freedom from addictions, emotional scars, mental assaults, spiritual wounds, and social jealousies. Practical and biblical applications need to be the combined focus, not just an all-star exercise and nutrition plan with verses at the bottom of the page. The Holy Spirit led me to a penetrating component that we need God's plan, and not man's, to combat and defeat the enemy's attacks. I knew immediately I had to get women together to help build each other up.

My first step—I started a fitness class at church. After a few weeks, I realized meeting once per week with a devotional and a fitness class would not break us free from the torments on our health. We needed more accountability. I decided to pilot a fitness class with a small pamphlet that contained God-focused tools to help during the week—when we were not together. It was brief, but beyond what a mere fitness class offers. A lady in the pilot group who worked for the local newspaper told me I needed to publish this material. This was when the still small voice of the Holy Spirit surfaced in my mind. I didn't know if I should suppress it or welcome it. *Am I really author material?* As if ordained by God, another woman a few days later told me to publish this booklet, and she just happened to be a high school English teacher.

This little booklet soon expanded as those in the class pressed for more, which was when I acted and obeyed and took the first step. I pushed pause on my live classes and went to work on the actual book.

This was about the time the little devil on my shoulder, with doubt in one hand and negativity in the other entered my mind with force. *My English teacher told me I couldn't write. How am I supposed to write a book while raising my six children who are all in elementary school? When will I have time to make this worthy of publishing, among everything else I am involved in?*

A good friend's voice echoed in my mind: *He equips those He calls and doesn't always wait to call the equipped.* In training and under fire was to say the least as I began to work on it. With the start of each new week, I was immediately tested with each topic I introduced. I quickly figured out I could not write something if I did not walk the path myself. When I wrote on spiritual health, it was as if hell was unleashed and nothing went right. My kids were sick, cars broke down, our salaries decreased, and I questioned God. I walked in the shoes of whatever I penned for the next five years as I completed this book.

The Lord helped me press forward, along with spell-check, fabulous friends, and family. I never once felt alone. My personal walls came down, jealousies left, and fearful nights and worrisome days vanished as I prayed and grew closer to my Commander Jesus. I realized I needed to walk through these same battles before I could expect other women to jump in the race with me.

God gave me supernatural peace about the entire writing process. I learned to stop saying, "I'm not author material," and start saying, "I can do all things through Christ who gives me strength!" I prayed for a timeline of when to finish this book, so I could organize my publishing date and get this into the hands of others. No date was given. Leaving the whole thing up to God, I continued writing for the next few years as He cleared my schedule and multiplied my time.

As I neared the end of my writing, I needed someone to critique and edit. I prayed in the quietness of my room, *God please give me advice and direction. I'm floundering. Show me who to ask for help.* No more than three days passed and a friend walked up to me at church and said, "I know you are writing a book, and I'm not sure if you are close to being done, but I feel God wants me to help edit it." Flabbergasted by how quickly God answered my prayer,

I was most intrigued by God's irony. The woman just happened to be a stay-at-home mom who recently retired from being a high school English teacher.

The journey from the first whisper in my heart some 20 years ago is filled with many amazing God-moments. In fact, as I sought out a final rough draft editor, God went before me and beautifully orchestrated my steps once again. You will read this story in the book; she's my sidewalk lady! He can do outstanding things in our lives if we are patient and open to His plans—and not rely on our own. This book is a life-changer for me, and I know it will be for you. It is based on God's plan, not some crazy busy woman who thought it would be a good idea to publish a book.

I'm so excited for your journey! I prayed for YOU, yes YOU, before your hands ever touched this book. This whole process of writing a book reminds me of the story of Esther (It's a fabulous read) on how God led her to where and when she needed to be—exactly how God planned. Even though God lined up all the details for her, Esther still had to engage physically and do her part. It was hard, scary, and laced with emotional and mental barriers, but these circumstances set her up to be one of the most courageous leaders in the Bible.

Esther was a woman, just like you. She wasn't made out of anything other than what you are made of. What made her different from most was obedience. She had a calling on her life, just as you have on yours. God is calling you to do things for Him because you have life purposes. Do you hear His voice? Do you know what He is calling you to do this week, next week, or next year? I believe you were meant to pick this book up and take this journey. I believe you are here (on this earth) for such a time as this (Esther 4:14).

PROGRAM SETUP AND PRE-EVALUATION

Identifying Accountability Partners

There are countless women dragging through life as they stand cornered with huge health battles—alone and afraid. They need you, and you need them. Having a strong and available support system is the key component to advance in battles, big or small. This book is a journey and to be experienced together with someone else. Prayerfully consider who should accompany you for the next 14 weeks on your journey.

God gave you special girlfriends to uphold, love, stand beside, be accountable to, and even with whom to walk through the craziness of this world. God knows women need to talk (some more than others), listen, cry, laugh, and love. He created us this way. However, there is truth that you connect better with some women than others. Ask God to help you decide if you are to run this race with just one woman or in a small group.

At times, this journey will ask difficult personal questions, some of which could take you to the Grand Canyon of your soul. Hidden health concerns could surface as conversations go deeper before climbing to mountain peaks. Let yourself in on this secret: you do not have to keep any super-woman title. Be real, be honest, and be you. This will be a give-and-take journey. One week you may be the encourager and the next, the encouragee. This is why it is vital to connect with God first and pray for direction with whom to share these special moments. I have faith that you can find and connect with at least one of the billions of amazing women God created.

There are three degrees of accountability you can encounter on this journey:

Accountability with God. Being accountable to God can look different to everyone. Ask God:

- What being accountable to Him looks like for you personally.
- To give you daily time to pray.
- Questions, and wait for answers.

Accountability Partner (AP). AP attributes should have qualities attractive to you. Who will be:

- Open with honest communication.
- Accountable with you, without getting upset.
- Available at the frequency you need.
- Trustworthy and have the ability to keep conversations private.
- Available to pray with and for you.

Accountability Group (AG). You may have the privilege of going through this book in a small group with your AP. For example, if another set of APs meets with you and your AP, this would create a small accountability group. Another option is to have three in a small group if there is not a fourth AP.

Note: *Read the Accountability Group Details on the next page.*

Accountability Group Details

If you have the option to meet as an accountability group while going through this program, consider yourself truly blessed. There are two different types of accountability groups you may encounter.

Small Accountability Groups are up to 4 people and can be formed with two sets of APs.

1. These small groups meet together on a weekly basis.
2. Please limit your AG to 4 women—it keeps the group intimate and allows more personal information to be shared.
3. If the group seems too big, even if you are already half way through this book, form another group.

Large Accountability Groups are a gathering of small AGs that all meet together at the same time and place.

1. These larger groups encourage accountability for each of the small AG's.
2. These groups are very helpful if AG's would like to exercise together.
3. In order to organize a large AG gathering, start by choosing an AG SEL (Simple Encouraging Lady) Leader. An SEL leader's role could include:
   - Setting up dates, times, and securing a location with adequate space for the size of the group.
   - Facilitating by opening and closing in prayer, timing the meeting length, setting up possible childcare and group exercises/videos if needed.
   - Helping suggest placement of women for small AGs if necessary.

Please Note:
An AG is not a strict and stringent group. It is aimed to be a support and accountability gathering for women to share their triumphs and trials in a trusting and loving place, sharing freely—not regurgitating answers to questions. Allow fellowship and lots of it, but be mindful of the needs of others in your group.

The Basics of the Course

Your whole-person health journey with your AP or AG will last 14 weeks. Not every group will travel the same path, so you and your accountability partner(s) get the chance to set some of the course details together.

After you decide on this crucial part of your journey—identifying an AP or AG—the second decision is what day, time, and place you want to meet together for your weekly accountability time. It is during these meetings that you will bond in a beautiful way as you review the devotionals you digested during your personal time that week. You will also have the opportunity to exercise together, utilizing plans given in the second week. I wholeheartedly believe that girlfriends who pray and exercise together stay together!

Book Setup

This journey will point to the Armor of God in Ephesians 6 and will relate it to various areas of our health. There are seven sections to this book. Each section contains two weeks. The first week in each section focuses on a piece of God's armor. The second week in each section targets the complementary health component. Take the entire week to digest the material successfully. You will have the opportunity to meet with your accountability partner(s) at the end of each week. Since there are 14 weeks, you will meet 14 times. **Do not meet until after you have read Week 1.**

Armor Alert

These sections are key encouragements and challenges that should not be skipped. Use intention. These Armor Alerts are what you will review with your AP/AG every week on your indicated meeting day.

Treasure Chest

This special section is located in the back of the book and contains exercise plans with progressions and modifications, charts, fit recipes, easy to follow meal plans, and more.

Physical Training Program

This health journey is not just about exercise; in fact, exercise is only about 20 percent of your overall health. You may already have access to a personal trainer, 20 exercise videos, a local gym membership, a rowing club, or indoor fitness equipment. Be a good steward of these healthy avenues and enjoy your community with others as much as possible. Week 2 will go through other options for exercise and modifications (a word that allows any fitness level to exercise).

The Armor of God

The below verses are the basis for the entire book. Read them and internalize them, even if you have read the passage many times before.

> "Finally, my brethren, be strong in the Lord and in the power of His might. Put on the whole armor of God, that you may be able to stand against the wiles of the devil. For we do not wrestle against flesh and blood, but against principalities, against powers, against the rulers of the darkness of this age, against spiritual hosts of wickedness in the heavenly places. Therefore take up the whole armor of God, that you may be able to withstand in the evil day, and having done all, to stand.
>
> Stand therefore, having girded your waist with truth, having put on the breastplate of righteousness, and having shod your feet with the preparation of the Gospel of peace; above all, taking the shield of faith with which you will be able to quench all the fiery darts of the wicked one. And take the helmet of salvation, and the sword of the Spirit, which is the Word of God; praying always with all prayer and supplication in the Spirit, being watchful to this end with all perseverance and supplication for all the saints—and for me, that utterance may be given to me, that I may open my mouth boldly to make known the mystery of the Gospel, for which I am an ambassador in chains; that in it I may speak boldly, as I ought to speak."—Ephesians 6:10-20

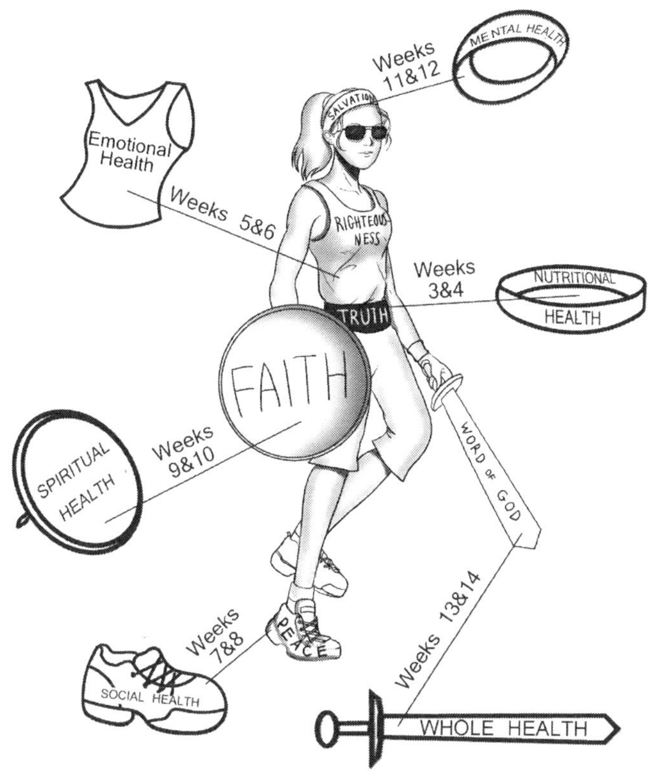

The Pre-Evaluation: A Snapshot of Your Overall Health

The following chart shows different health areas. These areas of health will be the focal points in your journey. They are listed in the order you will find them in this book and are broken down into two-week sections. Take a few honest minutes to look at your current health by answering these questions. There is no answer key and no right or wrong answers because you are personally evaluating yourself. You may already distinctly know which health area you exceed. My prayer is that you will be as honest as you can to experience growth through this health journey.

1. **Underline attributes you love about yourself from the right boxes.**
2. **Now repeat this action step on the left side and underline areas you would like to experience more growth.**
3. **Look at both sides of the chart and place an X on each arrow indicating where you fall closest to, the right side box or the left side box.**
4. **Using the arrows as your indicator, which one health area** (physical, nutritional, emotional, social, spiritual, or mental) **does the X fall closest to the right—the area you feel strongest?**
5. **Why do you feel strong in these areas? Go ahead and brag about yourself!** (The underlined words will help.)
6. **Which one health area does the X fall closest to the left—the area you feel needs the most growth?** (This is the first health area you will focus on as you being your journey.)
7. **Why? Why do you desire more growth in these areas?** (The underlined words will help.)

The Pre-Evaluation chart is based on the truths found in the Bible. Romans 1:20 tells us God's invisible attributes are clearly seen, that He is in charge of creation and that no one will have an excuse that she did not know God existed when she perishes. If God is our creator, then His Word, the Bible, is truth. His Word clearly states what is good and what is not, and for what we should strive and from what we should steer clear.

Finish the question: I am …

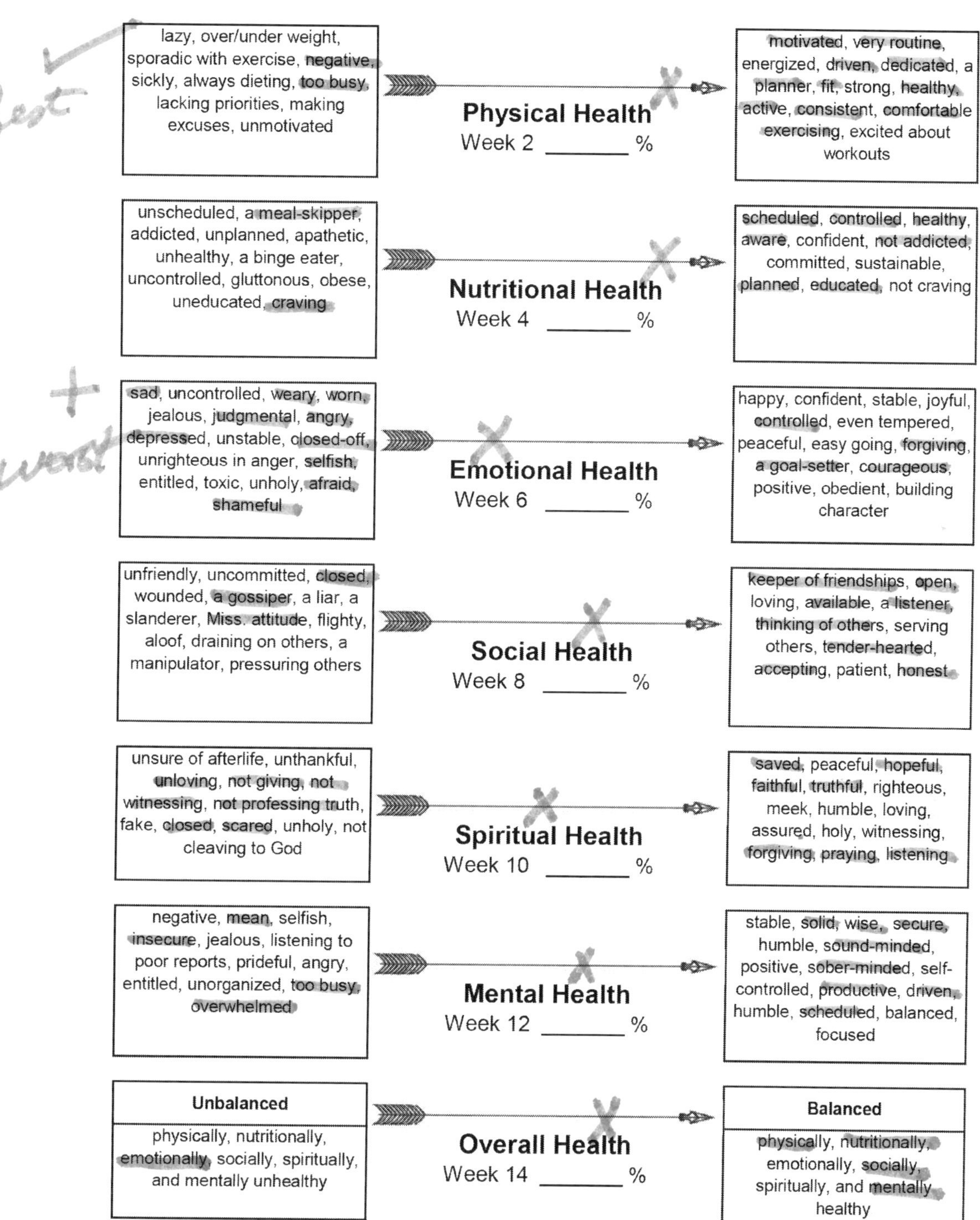

"Let all bitterness, wrath, anger, clamor, and evil speaking be put away from you, with all malice. And be kind to one another, tenderhearted, forgiving one another, even as God in Christ forgave you."
—Ephesians 4:31-32

SECTION ONE

THE WAR ON YOUR HEALTH

Even though a rock-solid nutrition plan and the latest training program are the most common goal-setting avenues for health and highly targeted every January, they are not the best way to go about overall health. There is something much more destructive to our health that we should place our focus—the inner negative struggle.

This internal struggle (battle, negativity, voice) goes back to the beginning, a day we are familiar with when the shamelessly naked couple in the Garden of Eden took the ultimate test. A tricky serpent lured his way into Eve's mind by whispering nonsense about how she did not need to obey God, that she could look from "within" to gain wisdom, and that *her* decisions were much better than God's. Because she listened and processed the negative information, the lie took root in her heart, and soon her mental, social, and physical health changed forever. This serpent, named Satan in the Bible, quickly deceived her into his invisible rebellion of self, the "I."

This successful act was of ultimate deception because sin's disastrous consequence became universal; no one became excluded. You and I from birth were grandfathered into this self-serving "I." This moment in time placed all of creation at odds with God and itself. Even though this unrest is all spiritual in nature and is an unseen battle within our minds, it opened the door to a significant decline that placed a bull's-eye on our health today. *Ladies, we are in the middle of this invisible battle regardless if we accept the invitation to join or not.*

Genesis 3 depicts many things lost due to this Fall of man—dominion over the earth, satisfaction, peace, and harmony in marriage to name a few. Not only did our workloads become laborious (especially with birthing), the physical earth became a dying world that plagued and aged animals, plants, and all living things—including us. *Without the Fall we would not have wrinkles!* Instead of a thriving, everlasting world, it became one with disease and death. This spiritual unrest is deep. It is nothing I naturally want to be a part of. It is something I do not wish on anyone, but it's too huge to ignore. This downfall granted more ramifications on our physical bodies than just wrinkles. It gave birth to a spiritual battle on our health, all perpetuated by the enemy's deceitful voice, which anchored in the open ear of one who listened.

The first week of this section opens our eyes to this battle and how it is affecting us. Just because we don't want to read or talk about this side of our health doesn't mean it's nonexistent. We each have struggled at one point or another with our health—even if mental or emotional. God gave us a plan, and a means to silence the negative struggle and win our health battles. The second week compliments the first by offering an action plan focused on physical health.

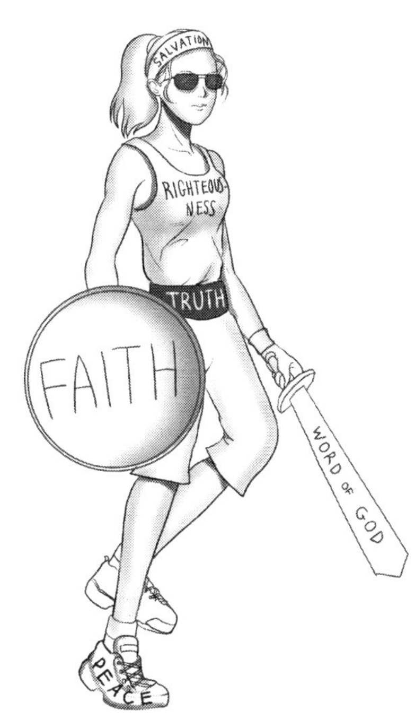

Week 1: Preparing for Battle
Week 2: Arm Yourself with Physical Health

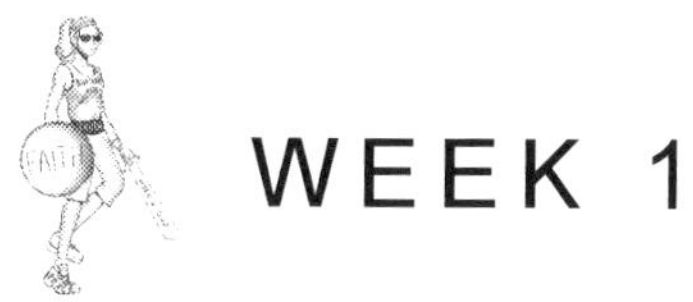

WEEK 1

PREPARING FOR BATTLE

Week 1, Day 1
Accepting the Spiritual War

"For we do not wrestle against flesh and blood, but against principalities, against powers, against the rulers of the darkness of this age, against spiritual hosts of wickedness in the heavenly places."
—Ephesians 6:11–12

I knew there was a spiritual side of things out there and accepted it, but I never realized I had anything to do with it. I was misled to believe it was too intangible to entangle me. I thought if I left all that spiritual stuff alone that it would leave me alone. I had myself convinced *I* was doing a good job with my little paper swords—the means by which I fought my health battles. After all, I had fabulous willpower and if I put my mind to it, I could do almost anything.

And this is where it all went wrong.

I didn't realize how much the enemy was truly on the prowl, trying to sabotage my health, of all things—and at such a deep level. This adverse and jealous whisper war became more destructive to my health. The voice of negativity got worse when it suggested I ponder and react in ways I thought I would never even consider. *Why is she so special? You have nothing on her. You are so much better than that group of ladies.*

It was evident to me I could not fight these whispers, voices, battles, or whatever was raging within me. These invisible forces were no match for my arsenal of defense—especially my measly, ineffective willpower.

Some of us do not give merit to these harmful invisible forces that war against us. Instead, we accept Karma, accept action/reaction, do not believe these little devils even exist, or just ignore the whole issue because it is uncomfortable. When we fail to recognize there is an opposing side trying to destroy us, we take things personally when hurt or attacked by others. We revolt, get even, seek revenge, or remain bitter against people who mistreat us. These thinking, acting, and emotional charges make us engage in the wrong war.

We war against our bodies. We try to eat better and restrict calories or starve ourselves and become miserable. We run more, join more fitness classes, and tax our bodies. We can never seem to catch up. Our willpower just does not have enough to win. We do not have enough in us to win alone. We need God to fuel us, recharge us, mentor us, renew us, and lead us. If we had everything we needed and were perfect, why would we need Him? We are in a battle and need our Commander in Chief. We need to follow a plan and stand firm in our hope and faith in Him, even with things as seemingly insignificant as our food choices.

All this warring in the secret invisible place is very real and alive. It truly can be a fearful thing. It is weird to read about it, talk about it, or even think about it too much. But this is more than an angel on one shoulder and a tiny devil with a pitchfork on the other, debating whether to make another trip to the buffet line. It is real spiritual communication with invisible forces that whisper lies. Reread the verse of the day. More than one antagonist is whispering to us. Countless forces of evil are waging war, and it's not just flippant suggestions to make us fail at our health goals. They attack our entire being.

An inner beckoning suggests we do things we do not want to do. It whispers things we do not want to hear. The voice comes from deceitful adversaries prowling around in secret places, seeking someone who will listen. Somehow these voices penetrate our minds and seemingly control our thoughts, which lead to actions. Casually, we tune in because the enigmas are too enticing to shut out, which gives Satan his foothold.

"Diet and exercise are not the sources of our lagging health battles. We are focused on the wrong war."

We have all allowed this negative voice to quietly penetrate our hearts and minds. These thoughts for me started out simple enough. *Eat another basket of chips and salsa. Sleep in, and don't exercise today. Since you already had four brownies, what's one more?* In honesty, diet and exercise are not the sources of our lagging health battles. We focus on the wrong war.

This war is beyond mustering up our willpower to try harder, stay on a particular diet plan, or determine in our minds not to be depressed today. *If only I could do this on my own.* We are failing because we are not armed properly to fight these foul and deceitful voices. This downfall has us females battling the wrong enemies—each other, God, and ourselves.

God provides a means to combat the enemy and his evil following so we can progress in our life journey with excellence—the Armor of God

ARMOR ALERT: Surrendering Your Paper Swords

It is time to lay down any paper swords—the means by which you currently stave off, ignore, or fight your battles. Maybe your paper sword is your mouth, time, selfishness, ill thoughts, unbelief, or even your lunch box. Whatever the habit, the desire, the feeling, the hurt, the addiction, or the entitlement you are currently using to combat the "I," here is your chance to allow God to have it and give you rest. So relax. You can overcome so much more with God leading you.

1. **Look back at the Pre-Evaluation chart and identify a few specific underlined words (from the left side) you battle with the most.**

SAD WEARY, WORN OVERWHELMED
ANGRY/ SELFISH

2. **What godly attributes do you feel you lack (such as love, faith, joy, peace, patience, faithfulness, gentleness, self-control, meekness, holiness, commitment, dedication, strength, forgiveness, hope, assurance of salvation, prayer, kindness, or acceptance)?** JOY HOPE PATIENCE

3. **How would the attributes you lack in question 2 be a possible solution to the areas you battle with in question 1?**

If I had JOY & HOPE & PATIENCE I more than likely wouldnt feel SAD WORN WEARY OVERWHELMED & ANGRY

 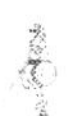

Week 1, Day 2
Summoning Sooner

"There are two equal and opposite errors into which our race can fall about the devils. One is to disbelieve in their existence. The other is to believe, and to feel an excessive and unhealthy interest in them."
—CS Lewis

When one of my children is sick, I diagnose the problem: fever, head cold, allergies, poor nutrition, etc. My assessment gives me as a mom the ability to better remedy, or at least help, the situation. One day it hit me, it seems that after my treatments fail, I revert to prayer. Conviction slapped me hard. I do not usually pray first. I guess with all these capable medicines; minor ailments seem like such a small thing with which to bother God.

As I read the New Testament Scriptures about people and their great faith—like friends taking off roof tiles to lower their crippled friend down to Jesus, a father asking Jesus just to say the words and his daughter would be healed, or a woman who thought if she could just touch His garment her blood disease would be relieved—I realized I too should come boldly to Him, no matter the so-called bother.

When Jesus was in His thirties, He was completely about His Father's business, walking the land and being followed by thousands. He had compassion for everyone He came in contact with, including those cast off from the community with leprosy. People were genuinely drawn to Him because He was fulfilling a deep need. Some were compelled by His teachings, His grace, His provision, and the love He so freely gave (like Mary Magdalena and His 12 disciples).

Jesus spent so much time healing others and freeing them from demons that there are too many instances to record in the Bible (John 21:25), which is further proof that the enemy has a direct target on our physical health. When our health suffers, we are debilitated from almost life itself. It can hinder and stop us from progressing in living a full-throttle life. People will do anything to be healed physically, as we read multiple times in the Bible.

We still struggle and battle with demons, disease, sickness, and the acceptance of God's Kingdom to this day. We do not physically see a lot of demonic activity in the Western world as much as in other countries. Possibly because we are doing such a good job just listening to the negativity and comparing ourselves to others that we don't need the same demonic activity other parts of the world experience?

It is not until we realize we are powerless to save ourselves and each other that we finally summon divine intervention. Someone more powerful must lead the way and fight with and

for us. God should be our starting point, not our last call when everything else we have tried fails.

Prayer is not listed directly as a piece of the Armor of God; rather it is the means by which we engage and fight the battle itself. When we pray, we are connecting with the King of Kings, the Creator of all, and are participating in spiritual warfare. We must arm ourselves with His spiritual armor. Our personal armor and paper swords have no effect while fighting the holy war. We cannot fight with physical means like trying to restrict food intake to win our health battles any more than we can throw a stick and wound a ghost. If we don't pray, we are not communicating with God. If we are not communicating with God, something else will communicate with us (1 Peter 5:8) and seek to destroy us.

"If we don't pray, we are not communicating with God. If we are not communicating with God, something else will communicate with us."

Even though we pray, it does not mean we will receive the answer we envision. God is not a vending machine. James 4 tells us we do not receive because we ask wrongly, to spend it on our passions. I know I have asked amiss in prayer, to please myself, the "I." We do not know why God heals some and not others, but we do know we can trust Him that His will and plan is better than ours—no matter how that makes us feel.

We know deep inside that something is different when we pray to the Almighty God. It is so much different then praying to a statue or shooting up a prayer indirectly to the air at no one in particular, hoping someone will hear. Prayer does not always have to be on our knees, on our face, or standing in a church service. It just has to be with Him.

ARMOR ALERT: Surrender

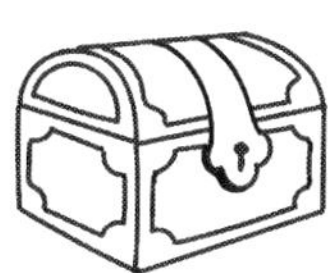

Some of us have already surrendered our lives to Christ, but might not be surrendering everything. If you have never surrendered your life to Him and would like to, or are ready to read more about it, please refer to the Treasure Chest in the section Surrender.

1. **Do you wait to pray until you have exhausted your own remedies? If so, why?**

2. **Since communication cannot be a one-time thing, when will you meet up with God next?** (Take a short coffee break and read Mark 5 for more on the cross between the spiritual and physical world.)

Week 1, Day 3
Scraping off the Wallpaper

"The Lord is near to all who call upon Him, to all who call upon Him in truth.
He will fulfill the desire of those who fear Him; He also will hear their cry and save them."
—Psalm 145:18-19

In a new state, purchasing an older house that had walls covered in wallpaper made me second-guess myself after signing the papers. Without the right tools, money, a lot of time, or friends to help, scraping it off surpassed the feat of physically running a marathon. I spent hours peeling, sanding, and crying with vivid frustration. *Why do people hang wallpaper in closets?* Just when I thought I was done, I uncovered some major cracks in the walls. In reality, we all hang wallpaper somewhere, masking something internally; we just hang different colors and styles and in various places.

I, for one, can easily hang wallpaper in the home of my mind. *What if they think less of me? I can't let others know I am insecure! I'm supposed to be the rock—they would know I'm weak.* It's hard to share shortcomings with others, so we pretend our imperfections do not exist as we construct walls here and there, and then hang lovely wallpaper all over them. It is even easier to build walls of justification when hurt. Consequently, the longer we hide behind our wallpaper it will just take that much longer to fix any real damage hiding underneath.

Our enemy is Satan, the fallen angel that wanted to be God, but never would, so he became the very thing God could not be. Not only have I been misled by the deceitful whispers from the enemy, too many times to count, as a fitness expert I have seen other women who followed suit. Some already had that perfect magazine figure, with an elegant exterior, but they too had cracked walls on the interior of their hearts and minds. They listened to those whispers: they were not strong enough, would never be truly beautiful, or did not measure up. It seems plausible that at the Fall, an extra dose of insecurity was bestowed upon the woman. Insecurity lowers our defenses and causes us to have that open ear to believe lies from deceitful whispers. It derails our thinking and illuminates our path to focus on all things opposite of God.

It is so important and necessary to connect with others who can help us scrape off wallpaper that is hiding cracks in our hearts. I may be able to admit I worry sometimes, but to admit to insecurity feels like standing naked at church—a very exposed feeling. On the contrary, the church is a perfect place to find such a friend to help heal vulnerabilities with trustworthiness, acceptance, and love. It is a body of believers, not just four walls with a steeple. The church's overall purpose is to give glory to God and make disciples of Jesus Christ and to encourage and build each other up in the faith while being the tangible hands and feet of Jesus.

In church, there are real people with real insecurities and real hurts. Some women long for others to bond, connect, share secrets, drink coffee, seek after Christ, and be accountable.

Real friends have real issues and will want you to be real with them. Consider taking down some wallpaper (allowing others to see the real you) and fixing some cracked walls underneath (admitting you are not perfect), or taking down the walls altogether (allowing help with an insecurity battle). It could be very scary, and incredibly humbling, but also freeing to finally fix something with the help of real friends. Friends are a blessing from God, as Proverbs 17:17 says, "A friend loves at all times."

The deceitful whisper tells the "I" to shut down friendships. The enemy wants us to remain childlike and ignorant of growth. He will do everything in his power to inhibit us from exposing a bare wall around our heart to our friends, which he convinces us will make us stronger and more powerful in the end. Sometimes he wins, and we decide not to share and take risks with this open friendship stuff. I can tell you a secret from experience. If we hide behind walls laced with wallpaper, we could miss some of the most amazing people God has strategically placed in our path. If we want to start winning this health war, we need to be real and stop pretending we have it all together. Friends know when we hide things, and so does God.

Women who get together and pray in Jesus' name have the confidence. The most important task is not merely to share and talk about our wallpaper, but to pray together on why the wallpaper went up in the first place (yes, another scary thing that happens in battle).

For some, praying may be as carefree as a walk in the park, but not all share this emotion. Praying together with someone can be as frightening as public speaking. Some have never prayed groups or out loud. I hear being nervous, sweating, and having heart palpitations are some side effects. Ponder this thought: if you are completely capable of conversation with one of your closest friends at any given time but become nervous when it's time to pray, this should absolutely give validity that you are in a spiritual battle. Something inside is setting off an alarm when people engage spiritually, so they hold back. Ask yourself if this happens to you.

Satan is going to try and withhold us from praying, especially together. He will plant whispers of doubt or lack of time, and he will continue plaguing us with insecurities. He will spew fear in our ears, lie that God will not listen, and tell us nothing will actually be answered. Stop the enemy's trash talk. You are stronger and more powerful with God as your advocate.

Talk to God as you would your best friend. Seek a friend to pray with you—like your AP. Spiritual engagement helps walls come down and your love of God going up. *Read Joshua and the battle of Jericho in Joshua 5-6—one of my favorite spiritual history lessons.

ARMOR ALERT: Accountability

Ladies, you are beyond beautiful and don't need wallpaper to make you pretty. Jesus loves you completely and at an unfathomable level. He wants to see you thrive in your life. Be you.

Be real. Be amazing. Your AP is here to encourage, challenge, and pray for and with you. Refer to the opening description of an AP in Program Setup and Pre-Evaluation, Identifying Accountability Partners, and refresh yourself on your role of being accountable to her.

1. **Decide what you will share about the pre-evaluation chart with your AP at your first meeting.** (How accountable can you truly be to her?)

2. **If you are not comfortable praying out loud, ask your AP for help. Practice before your meeting by using Jesus' words from the Scripture below as an example.** (Don't worry about the words you will say. It's like talking, and most women are excellent at that.)

> "In this manner, therefore, pray: Our Father in heaven, hallowed be Your name. Your kingdom come. Your will be done on earth as it is in heaven. Give us this day our daily bread. And forgive us our debts, as we forgive our debtors. And do not lead us into temptation, but deliver us from the evil one. For Yours is the kingdom and the power and the glory forever. Amen."
>
> —Matthew 6:9-13.

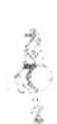

Week 1, Day 4
Courageous Commitment

"Commit thy works unto the LORD, and thy thoughts shall be established."
—Proverbs 16:3

I will never forget a specific youth conference that precisely changed the course of my life. The reason was simple—I made a public profession of faith in front of hundreds of other teenagers. It was a call to be obedient to whatever God called me to do. The first task was to physically get out of my seat, go to the front altar, and proclaim Christ in front of all the other teenagers. I know this was God calling me because I was beyond trembling inside, and my heart almost burst out of my chest. It is a feeling I only get when I know in my heart that I am supposed to do something for God. It goes beyond that gut feeling. I sometimes get goose bumps and above all, my heart pounds at irregular speeds—even if in the middle of a loud youth concert. This is how God sometimes spiritually communicates with me.

These physical reactions made me very aware of the spiritual battle warring inside as the negative voice tried to entice the "I" to make me physically stay in my seat. I showed God my desire to be obedient, and He gave me supernatural boldness to do so much more in the years to come. However, I do not always get it right. I still don't always answer God's call. Humility is kicking in here, but honestly, there are countless times I suppress the pounding because of pride or insecurity. I miss it most when I am listening too much to the "I," like those moments when I wake up specifically to pray, but something else seems to steal my time. I become busy with life. When this happens, it's like the negative voice gets louder as I listen more to myself, the "I," which jams communication with God.

When I am not communicating with Jesus daily, and I selfishly appease my own time, it is easy to drift slowly from Him. This fallen world pulls us away with so much force that it easily distracts us from the most important things in life. God wants to free us from our health battles, but He won't always do it when we are following someone else. He can save us years of anguish by overcoming the disobedience battle—obeying when we totally do not want to, when it does not make sense, and even when it hurts. God does not want us to fall prey to the negative inner dialogue as we grab another fistful of insignificant comforts. He challenges us to trust Him. That can require a courageous commitment to follow Him in a new area of our health.

I view commitment to mean being loyal to what you vowed long after the mood you said it in is gone. I encourage you to step out in faith and be courageous with your commitment. Today, you have the opportunity to commit the health of your entire body—physical, emotional, social, spiritual, and mental—to His call and not the "I."

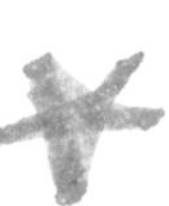

ARMOR ALERT: Commitment

This commitment is specific to this journey. Read through the preparation statements below and prayerfully consider your personal level of commitment before signing the pledge in number 7.

1. **Prepare Your Temple Physically** (Belt of Truth)
   Pray that God would help your physical body (specifically, name the areas you need the most help with—refer to your Pre-evaluation chart). The help might have to do with exercise or nutrition, but it may also be on a deeper level. Our bodies are instruments for good or bad. 1 Corinthians 6:18 says our body is a temple because the Holy Spirit resides in us. We must treat it like one. If you have sins hovering around the door of your heart, ask Christ to forgive you truly and to help you run from them.

2. **Prepare Your Heart Emotionally** (Breastplate of Righteousness)
   Pray and ask God to truly open your heart to His plans for your life, and then run after them (even if it means something crazy like writing a book or speaking in front of others). Ask Him to help you be honest and willing to take down any walls or wallpaper, and to humbly fill any cracks that need attention. "Being confident of this, that he who began a good work in you will carry it on to completion until the day of Christ Jesus" (Ephesians 1:6).

3. **Prepare Your Soul Mentally** (Helmet of Salvation)
   Allow God to transform your mind and erase poor thoughts and bad baggage, and to remove any poor self-images. Ask Him to help you understand and protect your salvation with daily renewal and connection with Him. "The mind governed by the flesh is death, but the mind governed by the Spirit is life and peace" (Romans 8:6).

4. **Prepare Your Relationships Socially** (Gospel of Peace)
   Ask God to help you honestly connect with your AP by allowing yourself to be raw (if you dare) and to be an encouraging and trustworthy AP yourself. Ask God to help you be a listener and not always the fixer (allow Him to do the fixing). Commit to being on time and prepared for every meeting. If it is hard for you to encourage others, ask God for help and wisdom, frequently. He will give it to you (James 1:5).

5. **Prepare Your Spirit Spiritually** (Sword of the Spirit)
   Make time to communicate with God—*with* is the key word. We can make time to pray, but maybe communication *with* God is spending time reading His Word (Sword of the Spirit) and listening with meditation. It is okay just to be still and silent (Psalm 46:10; Exodus 14:14).

6. **Choose a verse to memorize for this journey and write it below**. Choose a verse from today's reading, or another one you already know. Speak it daily and as much as possible. "Commit thy works unto the LORD, and thy thoughts shall be established" (Proverbs 16:3).

7. **Record below which area(s) God is calling you individually to commit to increasing in health during these following 13 weeks and how: physically, emotionally, mentally, socially, and spiritually.** I do believe as you walk through this journey, your particular area could alter and morph into another health area. This is natural. God could direct your steps in a new way, making one path lead to another. He promises us that when we seek, we will find if we search for Him with our whole heart.

"Commit your actions to the LORD, + your plans will succeed."
Pvbs 16:3

I will give my all and my very best to pursue excellence concerning my physical body, emotions, mind, spirit, and social relationships. I promise to encourage, communicate weekly, and pray for my Accountability Partner (AP) during this journey together.

____

My Signature *Date*

Ask your AP how she will commit to you, and then ask her to sign below at your first meeting together.

____

My AP Signature *Date*

Before You Meet

Deep, scared, timid, uneasy, excited, ready—these are feelings you can share at your first meeting with your AP/AG (this is one of the best parts of your journey)! Allow room for side conversations and sweet flowing fellowship. Your first meeting may be the longest. You will review your desires identified in your opening Pre-Evaluation Chart and discuss your most pressing answers and comments from Week 1. Review your week before you meet so you are ready to talk.

How is this first meeting supposed to go?

No Regurgitation, Please: This journey is not about answering questions and regurgitating them to someone else. Try to focus your conversation on the content of the week. Even if your conversation leads to little rabbit trails, don't shut down the conversation as long as it is God-focused and connected to the content.

Laugh: Remember to laugh a lot; it brings health to your bones.

Listen: If you are in a group setting, please take the time to listen and understand what others are communicating. Sometimes women need to share things but don't really want a solution—it just needs to be talked out. It can be a struggle when you hear something to not give advice, and to recognize that God may be allowing you to hear for a specific reason.

Trust: Be ready to share honestly. This is a no-shame zone. All women have highlights and hindrances and need a safe place to share with trust and love.

Encourage: At the end of every meeting, take turns and look each other in the eye. Share something amazing you see in her.

Share: Remember to review your opening chart first. Thumb through the week and decide which other specifics you wish to share.

IT'S TIME TO MEET!

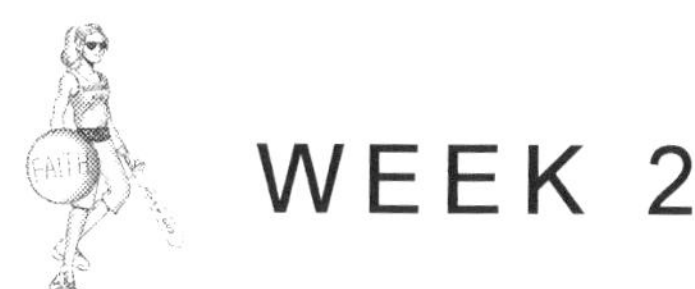

WEEK 2

ARM YOURSELF WITH PHYSICAL HEALTH

Week 2, Day 1
Fitness Organization

"The soul of the sluggard craves and gets nothing, while
the soul of the diligent is richly supplied."
—Proverbs 13:4, ESV

Imagine an Olympic swimmer or sprinter, NBA basketball player, or high school wrestler. Their fit bodies have very little fat and a distinctly chiseled form. Now think about a professional marathon runner. Their bodies are very thin with not nearly as much muscle mass as the above athletes for the number of hours they invest in their exercise routines. Both fitness-minded groups participate in at least one hour of exercise when they train. However, their bodies respond totally different to their selected training styles.

"Participating in sports or exercise is not what makes us healthy; it's the force behind it—discipline."

The type of exercise I enjoy most is weightlifting, however, sometimes what we like and what we actually get to do are different stories. In my thirties, I got injured and was limited to running, and I soon learned to enjoy it. Even after my injury healed, I became an avid racer. Just like the Olympic athletes, my body responded very differently to this new training style. I became very thin with little muscle (am excellent way to lose body fat). After a few years, I became bored with running and needed to add a little more muscle back on. I focused on interval training like the swimmers and sprinters. It allowed me to shorten my workouts so I could do other things I loved more.

I challenge you to test drive a few different training programs from the Treasure Chest, but first, I need to address the most common struggles. I am frequently asked how many times a week people should exercise and for how long. The answer is—it depends. For starters, what is your goal and how much time do you have to devote to exercise—and eating right? I exercise 45 minutes, four days per week, to maintain my body fat and muscle mass, and to be able to eat the way I want. The average person should exercise five times a week to lose body fat, but if a busy woman realistically only had three days to give, she could feel like a failure and quit. There is a solution for you personally, and my prayer is that you will find it. Regardless of what you do, make sure you do something. Participating in sports or exercise is not what makes us healthy; it's the force behind it—discipline.

Our time is precious, and we cannot seem to create enough of it. I cannot imagine living in the Wild West of the 19th-century when a man's average life expectancy was around 40 years. That is crazy short compared to Adam and Eve's longevity. We will make time for what is important. However, if we spend too much time on any one thing, we take time away from something else. We can squeeze in exercise anywhere at almost any time, and it does not need to take an hour a day.

Since our time is fleeting, as fast as gas in our tanks, we need a solid plan. The Bible tells us that people perish when there is no plan. "Commit your work to the Lord, and your plans will be established" (Proverbs 16:3). When organized with a health plan, we can commit it to God and ask Him for help. We can head into the day feeling prepared and more equipped to handle distractions. It is not that distractions do not come; it is that we are better prepared to handle them. For example, if you are at work and a package of donuts mysteriously appears in front of you, God can help you overcome the temptation of eating more than your coworker.

None of us knows the hour our last breath will be, so we cannot take one breath for granted, although it is easy to do. We can easily feel immortal and go about our daily living like tomorrow will always come. A heart attack, cancer, high blood pressure, and other diseases are called silent killers for a reason. They can take a life by surprise. James 4:14 reads, "Yet you do not know what tomorrow will bring. What is your life? For you are a mist that appears for a little time and then vanishes." This verse can seem depressing at first glance, but I see it as motivation. If we truly made the most of every encounter with others and lived our lives abundantly by asking God for the next new challenge, think how different we would live and enjoy our lives. Take each day as a gift, and make a lasting impact on those around you. It will bless you as well.

Following an exercise plan will keep us moving forward and make us feel like we will be here for another 100 years (I'm optimistic). The right exercise plan for you will allow more time on your plate for other things, and you'll see better results. When I stay active with exercise, I have more energy to do housework, I need less sleep, and I feel better in general. Being intentional with some energy output releases stress from our weary mindsets and bones, and results in increased mental clarity, so our brains excel with more productivity in less time. I have not met a woman yet that does not desire this.

ARMOR ALERT: Simple Planning

Discipline is necessary to achieve our goals, but equally important is accountability. Your AP is one of the best weapons you have to achieve your goals. You may already have a fantastic exercise plan. If this is true, you are among the few. This could be your week to share helpful nuggets with other women in your sphere of influence.

1. 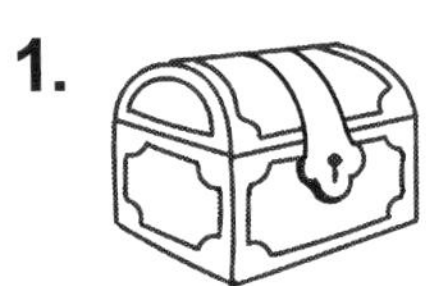 **Take a trip to the Treasure Chest and go to the section, Exercise Training Programs. Begin Step 1: Simple Planning. This may take a while pending your familiarity with exercise, so take your time, there is no rush to finish today.**

2. **After you are done with Step 1, at least begin Step 2: God's Fitness Tools. Read the different styles of training and ponder God's handiwork.** (He created your physical body with such complexities.)

Week 2, Day 2
Discipline Yourself

"For the moment all discipline seems painful rather than pleasant, but later it yields the peaceful fruit of righteousness to those who have been trained by it."
—Hebrews 12:11, ESV

I grew up playing the flute. I sure was not good at it when I started out, but after years of private lessons, and a tremendous amount of practice sessions, I conquered this area of discipline, and it paid my way through college. If I had only picked up my flute a few times here and there, I would never have been good. We can apply discipline to every area of our life: praying, cleaning, education, memorization, relationships, meal planning, exercising, and so on. But, have you ever thought we could apply discipline in areas that are not good? Of course, there are many areas I could admit to having discipline in that I am not so proud of, which is why I need God so desperately to direct my steps. Being honest, I had immense discipline in selfishness as I sat for almost an entire weekend to complete an fantastic TV series on Netflix. It would have been much more productive, and satisfying in the end, to have done just about anything else that weekend—especially since the ending was a total dive.

It takes an immense amount of discipline to reach the fitness level of an Olympic athlete. It is intimidating and admirable, but not everyone desires (or needs to desire) this level of physical effort. We all have different ideas, abilities, time, drives, passions, talents, and body shapes. However, there is a secret to being an elite athlete that we can all learn from, and an exceptional training program is not it. It is discipline.

"Discipline is not comfortable, but even so, it is absolutely needed to create excellence within us."

If the enemy wanted to attack our physical health, I would assume at least one fiery dart would be aimed at our discipline. I do not always want to eat healthy or go to the gym and exercise. It is also totally not fun to walk away from a beautiful chocolate masterpiece that everyone else is enjoying. But if this is part of my personal discipline to reach a health goal, I need to follow it. I do not gain muscle when I go to the gym and lift a few times, stop, and come back a few weeks later. I become stronger and maintain it when I continue in my exercise goals and eat healthy—discipline. Discipline is not comfortable, but even so, it is needed to create excellence within us. Discipline is not something that happens overnight. I'll be honest; it takes tons of hard work. This is exactly why we need God to give us strength from within. There are still times I struggle against following the selfish "I," as I believe we all will continue to do, at least from time to time, living in this fallen world.

What if you found out that your current disciplines were not that good for you after all, and you were actually wasting time, health, and energy? I have a friend who was charged by her physician to exercise and lose weight because of her diabetes. She decided to walk on a treadmill for about two hours every day (yes, incredible discipline). A few months later she went to her physician and was told she was not losing enough weight but was facing adrenal fatigue. She was devastated. Another friend joined a very expensive gym. They focused on power weightlifting. She loved it dearly, but her physician told her it was stressing out her body, that she was re-injuring herself, and that she needed to completely change her exercise. Both friends had extreme discipline in exercise but were going about it the wrong way. They wasted loads of time, health, and energy—too much energy.

The enemy can plant seeds all around us and make us feel we should do certain things, even though we should not. Ah, one of my favorite sayings—"Just because you can, doesn't mean you should." Just because everyone else is running a marathon, or everyone else is on a diet, or everyone else is volunteering, does not mean you should. All these things could distract us from God's plans for us, take our health down the wrong path, or make us miss something even more fabulous in the future. Ask God for help, listen to your body (it speaks to you all the time), and seek help from others before you jump in and give discipline to just anything, especially an exercise program that may be causing you more harm in the end.

With any decision, small or big, we should consult God first. Many times, I have made a decision that made sense in my mind to move forward with, but I knew in my heart something was off. This indeed was truly an internal battle (which stressed my physical health). Since my heart and my mind were at odds with the decision, my sleep suffered, and I returned to my old poor eating habits. Searching the Scriptures and praying helped me distinguish the right thing to do. When we meet up with Christ, sometimes in a quiet place, and just spend time listening, we can hear the answers best, even though sometimes it takes longer than we hope. These internal mental and emotional battles remind me so much of my struggle with nutrition and exercise.

Face it, most of us do not have a perfected plan when it comes to our physical health. We can quickly lose this battle in no time flat. It is as if discipline is good for our mind and emotions, but ultimately unattractive when it comes to restricting sweets, packaged foods, and a steady exercise routine. But when we keep to our plan of physical health, our bodies feel better, we can go the distance, do more in less time, think more clearly, and not be held up by constant sickness or lack of energy.

I like adventure racing, but I have friends that won't even consider it. I like cars, but I have no desire to race them, ever, yet I have friends who thrive on speed. God is so gracious that He gave each of us our own abilities, talents, dreams, and desires. This is a huge blessing, but because of the Fall of man in that ancient garden, sin turned it into a curse. We easily flock to secret desires that are ungodly, banquet tables that are beautifully laid out by the enemy—not intended for us by God. This is the war we are in, and the war we must fight with God's help.

Victory over our health battles will be so much more attainable with godly discipline and self-control. "A man without self-control is like a city broken into and left without walls" (Proverbs 25:28). "And whatever you do, in word or deed, do everything in the name of the Lord Jesus, giving thanks to God the Father through him" (Colossians 3:17, ESV). Not many can say they are more than conquerors in the categories of both nutrition and exercise. If you are among the mighty few, please take this time with your AP/AG to stand strong and encourage them, as your AP/AG might be returning the favor in the upcoming weeks. If you have not conquered either or both areas of your physical health, let's determine why.

ARMOR ALERT: Decisiveness

God made our inner beings with individual passions and desires, and we each reach for them in our own ways, regardless of how Satan tries to twist and sabotage them. It takes prayer and self-control to achieve and surpass some of our goals. Getting healthy is not easy for everyone, which is why people struggle with it. You can do all things through Christ who gives you the strength you need to attain your goals. Don't shut Him out of your journey. Bring Him along side you and ask for His guidance, encouragement, and help.

1. **What are your physical fitness/nutrition goals, or what is the picture of health you want to resemble?** (Large bulging muscles, slender and tone, thin, feeling healthy, looking healthy, being healthy, having more energy, being able to do more in less time, reducing cellulite, increasing longevity, stronger bones, a lower A1C, increasing range of motion, etc.)

2. **What do you believe is the greatest obstacle that may hold you back from achieving these goals?** (Time, self-control, determination, dedication, purpose, reason, peace, education, accountability, health, family, planning, etc.)

3. **How could the answer to question two be a possible solution to the answer in number one?**

4. **If you didn't have the time yesterday to read the section, Exercise Training Programs, Step 2: God's Fitness Tools, please read through the parts that are most intriguing to you.**

Week 2, Day 3
Goldilocks

"He gives power to the faint, abundant strength to the weak. Though young men faint and grow weary, and youths stagger and fall, they that hope in the LORD will renew their strength, they will soar on eagles' wings; They will run and not grow weary, walk and not grow faint."
—Isaiah 40:29-31

Some of my younger daughters are new to social media. They are slowly getting accounts as we allow (and as their maturity seems ready for). These accounts are like our bathroom scales; they can hinder as much as they can help. A few weeks ago my seventh grader said there was a milk challenge going around on-line and asked if she could try it. The challenge was to drink one gallon of milk in one hour without throwing up. I told her indeed it was a challenge, but not a good one. People can drink milk, but they need a balance. My favorite saying, "Just because you can, doesn't mean you should." *I did not allow her to try this challenge.*

Back in the day, almost everyone needed to use physical brawn to till the land. Even children worked hard physically. This, of course, expelled energy and calories, just by yielding their very own food supply. They did not sit around at a desk and eat casually when they were hungry—or bored. In today's age, it is no secret that we consume too many calories and do not burn them all off in one day. This is why our culture is flooded with many different challenges and diets. Too many calories by the time we hit the pillow at night add extra cellulite on our butts, thighs, bellies, and even around our hearts. Too many days of this in a row leads to internal health issues. This in turn can become a habit or addiction. Balance truly is the new *real* challenge.

For those of us who do not till the land or burn calories in our daily duties, we need to find an outlet to perform an energy expenditure, or the laws of nature will trump. We could always eat less packaged foods and eat more healthy choices, but we all know that is not as easy to do in this super-sized fast food society. If you happen to be among the few who are naturally thin, you should also perform a physical activity so your muscles do not wither, and your bones do not become brittle. Think Goldilocks—not too much or too little, but just right. Having balance in our life is a very wholesome approach.

According to 1 Timothy 4:8, "Physical training is of some value, but godliness has value for all things, holding promise for both the present life and the life to come." Godliness is supposed to have the most value in our lives. It is useful for the present and the future. This means exercise should not be our focus, but should not be neglected either—Goldilocks. Godliness is profitable for all things, even our physical health. We should devote our attention to God and how He can fuel us internally—emotionally, socially, spiritually, and mentally, and not just our nutrition and exercise.

> **"When wealth is lost, nothing is lost; when health is lost, something is lost; when character is lost, all is lost."—Billy Graham**

Godliness means many things to many people, but mainly, it means to become more like Christ every day. We can have godliness in our emotional health (the way we righteously respond) and in our mental health (the way we process and value salvation). We can have godliness in our social health (the way we love and show peace to others) and in our spiritual health (the way we live out and demonstrate our faith). All these areas should be balanced in our lives, but I for one can be bombarded quickly. The attention on one outweighs the attention on the others at times. If we geek out with some general math for just a bit, evaluating the areas of our health in percentages, we can see if we place too much of our energy in one area.

20% Physical Health
20% Nutritional Health
20% Emotional Health
20% Social Health
20% Spiritual Health
20% Mental Health
100% Whole Health

The evenly balanced percentages in this chart should remind you of the Pre-Evaluation chart. Giving God our focus and obedience while we glorify Him in our heart, works, service, relationships, spirit, and the physical body is all part of His whole health plan for us. We may never have these balanced out at the "20 percent" mark, and honestly, they shouldn't be. There isn't a perfect equation for these percentages because we all have different battles that will take our focus off one area and place it on others. I may struggle with lack of exercise because my season of raising a family uses up that time. The point is not to stay unbalanced forever and be aware to squeeze it in a little, even if it's at a measly two percent (that's better than zero).

We cannot neglect eating well, or the laws of nature will trump (heart attack, obesity, clogged arteries, disease, lack of energy, etc.). Our nutrition is like a savings account. We may not feel the effects until it's too late. It all comes back to balanced living—Goldilocks.

The average person should not engage in heavy exercise every day of the week but should have some sort of activity. The smarter we exercise, the more time and energy we will have for other important aspects of our life. What if we sat in a chair and read our Bible all day, and never implemented what it told us to do—like making disciples? If we were astounding in our mental capacity and could recite and explain any passage of Scripture, but were not loving in our speech, the Scriptures say we would be like a creaky, rusty gate.

Since we are talking percentages, look at the chart below *(I know it's a little nerdy to break things down on a mathematical level).* Take our physical health percentage. An effective workout may only last 25 to 45 minutes, 3 to 4 times per week. For the average person, planning meals, preparing food, and actually eating during the day should take more time than planning and implementing our exercise regimes. Our nutrition should take more time than our exercise. It's that important.

Put it together:
Physical Health = 20% (4% Exercise + 16% Nutrition)

Most of us could use improvement somewhere in our physical health, either exercise or nutrition (*thanks to sitting at desks and our fast-food society).* Our bodies were created to move. Some cardio routines and training programs are 20 minutes and prove better results than an hour of treadmill running. I know some mothers who cherish their hour of alone time and take every moment on that treadmill, but take some of that time to even out exercise routines with stretching, balance, and weight training with tubes, bands, weights, balls, or bodyweight. Arming yourself with fitness in a variety of methods is one key to achieving a truly physically fit body.

ARMOR ALERT: Focus

Think about the effort you give to certain areas of your health. Is your focus unbalanced or just about right? Maybe you need to give more than 20 percent in a certain area, such as physical health in preparation for running a half marathon this year. Only you know what actually needs more focus over another area. The real question here is—are these areas balanced for you?

1. **On a scale of 1-100%, what percentage would you assign each category personally for yourself?**
   40 % Physical Health: Exercise & Nutrition
   15 % Emotional Health: Character & Emotions
   15 % Social Health: Family & Relationships
   20 % Spiritual Health: Love & Righteousness
   10 % Mental Health: Intelligence & Obligations
   = 100 % Whole Health

2. **Now fill these percentages in on your Pre-Evaluation Chart from the beginning on the blank lines by the titles.**

3. **Whatever your various percentages, what do these results show you personally?**

Too much focus on 1 area & the rest of my life is falling apart

 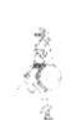

Week 2, Day 4
The Comparison Scale

"I appeal to you therefore, brothers, by the mercies of God, to present your bodies as a living sacrifice, holy and acceptable to God, which is your spiritual worship. Do not be conformed to this world, but be transformed by the renewal of your mind, that by testing you may discern what is the will of God, what is good and acceptable and perfect."
—Romans 12:1-2

I need to come clean with you all, and it is quite humbling. I have walked into a room, seen a woman that I didn't even know, and immediately disliked her, not because she wasn't cute, smart, or funny, but because she was too perfect looking. Not only did I not know her, I honestly did not want to. How crabby, prideful, selfish (and a whole bunch of other bad names I can think to call myself) was I? The "I" was too busy comparing myself to her. I never even gave her a chance to be my friend.

The verse at the top reminds us to keep focused on Christ by renewing our minds. There is a reason why we need to do this daily. Someone is trying to make us choose not to be Christ-like. It goes back to the deceitful whisper that suggests someone is better than us and that we should retaliate against the one who is showing us up.

It is so easy to be sucked into the thoughts and patterns of this world when we are not talking to God often. We want to be accepted, needed, and valued, and when we do not talk to God, we go looking for it elsewhere. We can size-up with airbrushed women in magazines, the perfect flat-abs-20-something, and the no-love-handles mom at the beach all because of this invisible comparison scale—the level we expect to achieve. This misconception masterpiece is the enemy.

Our thoughts can bog us down with trying to live up to something we will not achieve, can not achieve, or that our husbands do not even really want us to achieve. The secular viewpoint comes from the enemy who has the world convinced we need to weigh a certain number, have a certain chest size, and keep our thighs looking a particular way. The world misleads us into believing people are valued by the way they look—it is all a big whopping lie!

Christ provides freedom from all the mind muck of comparison and conformity. We will never fit in every social group on earth because we are not from here. We are sojourners passing through. John 15:19 writes that we are not of the world and so the world *hates* us (very strong verbiage here). Why do we try to please people who do not like or know us? No woman I know wants to feel hated by others. In an effort for people to cherish us, we choose to please the "I" and selfishly try to outdo others physically, mentally, and socially.

One of the grandest enemies with trying to look perfect or attain a certain body weight is the scale itself. This little device can very well hinder as much as it can help. Many women hop on a scale every day and allow it to control their very life. If they gain a half pound one day, they dive into a depression that wrecks their day before it even starts. Sure, the scale can help show progress, but there are a few little secrets when it comes to the scale we must be aware of.

Five pounds of feathers equals the same as five pounds of rocks, yet they take up space differently. Muscle and fat weigh the exact same, but they too look very different under our skin. As adults, we need to keep as much muscle as possible because our bodies are losing muscle and bone density (another uplifting aspect as our body ages). The more muscle we have in our bodies, the more calories we burn to maintain that muscle at rest. There are many benefits of gaining muscle: stronger bones, more energy, faster recovery from illness, and ability to perform daily tasks better—all of which will improve the quality of life. Another little secret—it takes time to lose body fat. The television shows that depict losing 10 pounds repeatedly every week are Hollywood in its glory.

I do not personally own a scale because I regulate my health based on the way I feel and the way my clothes fit. I do not want my five daughters, who all have different body shapes, to think there is a magic number they need to attain to be healthy.

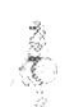

ARMOR ALERT: Attention Habitual Weighers

My son's teacher asked his class to track how many times they checked their phones in an eight hour period. One student checked it over 150 times. I trust no woman is hopping on the scale that much, but there seems to be an arrow pointing at it, encouraging us to jump on. Habitual weighing is a hindrance and an addiction that we can easily break if we set our mind on what matters.

1. **Do not weigh yourself until your last week of this book. Place a post-it note on the scale that reads STOP, hide it in the closet, give it to a friend, or just pitch it. Trust God and yourself. You are not identified by a number. Ask yourself how you feel instead of asking the scale.** (God wants you to connect with Him more than you are connecting with the scale.)

2. **Likewise, trash magazines or delete any social media avenue that would make you compare yourself to others.**

3. **Move forward in the Treasure Chest with the Exercise Training Programawms, Step 3: Choose Your Level of Fitness. This is a very packed out section with many options for exercise. I trust you will use this chest of treasures for years to come.**

Trainer Talk

I hope your second week of this journey was enlightening. The Treasure Chest is packed with exercise opportunities. I encourage you to try as many as you can—at your own pace of course. Don't worry if you aren't able to perform all the plans. I'm just excited for you to look through them and learn different exercise options. Share with your AP one new exercise you are going to try.

Our identity is in Christ, not in how other people view us.

Testimony

Christmas 2012—the towel read "because I am committed," a reminder from my family of where I began almost four years earlier—with a promise to them that I would get healthy. That meant I needed to get moving. I weighed 320 pounds. Ouch. I cried. I did not know how much work and time would be involved. I was so fearful I couldn't keep that promise. I had never made myself accountable to anyone but myself, and I always failed and never finished.

Negative thoughts filled my mind. *You're 53 years old. It's been 30 years. Why try again?* I would wake up and go to sleep wishing and hoping, dreaming and praying about losing weight. I needed my mind to be free. I knew what God's Word said in Romans 6:6—consider (reckon—believe in faith) to be dead to sin but alive to God. Did I really believe that? That I'm dead to sin? *Lord, help me in my unbelief.* Faith means action, so I began walking, eating better, and I hired a trainer (for strength and accountability). God's amazing peace sustained me. After a year, I lost 107 pounds. I was in constant awe of Him.

You know that fear I had? It immobilized me. Kept me in bondage. God has tenderly shown me it was not my commitment to my family (that would be a work of my own) that set me free. The truth is, as a child of God, He has always been committed to me. So that towel that was given to me could read "because I AM committed."

Barb Kuhl
Eldridge, Iowa

Before You Meet

Before you meet with your AP or AG, look over this page and truly ponder and take it all in.

Consider the Physical Health portion of your Pre-Evaluation Chart for a moment. Do you have a better understanding of how to move from the underlined words on the left side of this chart to the right?

<u>Left side of chart</u>: lazy, over/under weight, sporadic with exercise, negative, sickly, always dieting, too busy, lacking priorities, making excuses, unmotivated

<u>Right side of chart</u>: motivated, very routine, energized, driven, dedicated, a planner, fit, strong, healthy, active, consistent, comfortable exercising, excited about workouts

The spiritual war going on in the unseen world is bigger than we can imagine. The enemy does not want you to pray with someone else. He will try to thwart your plans to pray together as he fills your mind with doubt, insecurity, poor memories, fears of failure, or a desire not to meet. Knowing this, place those fears behind you and arm yourself with God's truths you learned these past two weeks.

Week 1—Prepare for Battle Review: Remember to ask God to help put away your paper swords and to fill you with His attributes. Go to Him first instead of waiting until later. Surrender to Him and ask God for the courage to pray with your AP/AG and share your most pressing thoughts and answers.

Week 2—Arm Yourself with Physical Health Review: This week should have given you some ideas to promote your physical exercise to the next level—having a plan, making the time, balancing your schedule, and establishing the discipline to focus on God's image of you.

After you have prayed and discussed this week with your AP, tell her something amazing about her. Don't forget to laugh. It is so good for your soul!

IT'S TIME TO MEET!

SECTION TWO

BELT OF TRUTH

Roman soldiers were well-trained and equipped to engage in war at a moment's notice. They valued their armor and weapons and knew the importance of each piece in battle. One of the essential pieces a soldier would put on was his belt, because that is where the rest of his armor connected and weapons resided. God, through Paul, cleverly used this metaphor of a belt to instruct us to gird ourselves with truth. We are in a spiritual war, which means we must be armed with spiritual weapons in order to fight. Truth is the first weapon listed in the Armor of God. Truth is extremely powerful and essential in our battles. We must attach it to us at all times—because without it, everything would fall apart.

We desperately need God in our battles spiritually, just as we desperately need food to keep us living physically. Food is analogous with God, and we should desire God as much as we desire to satisfy our hunger. He should be our daily bread (Matthew 6:11). Physically speaking, just as a belt surrounds our stomachs, so too should good nutrition. This is why the belt of truth and nutritional health complement each other so nicely, and why we will compare the need for both in these next two chapters.

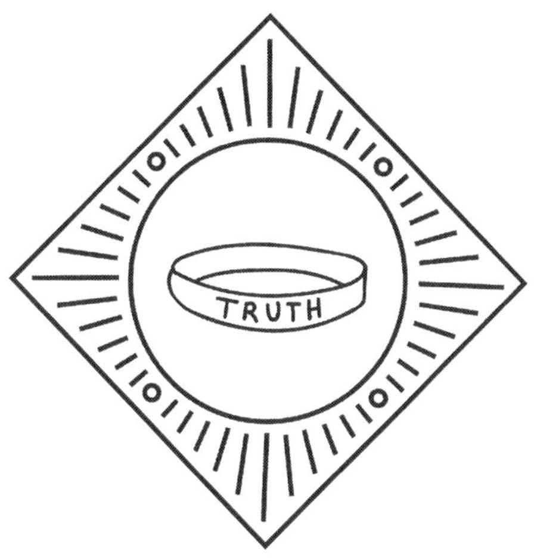

Week 3: Arm Yourself with Truth
Week 4: Arm Yourself with Nutritional Health

Health Challenge #1
2-Week Nutrition Challenge

Below is a list of a variety of nutrition challenges. For the next two weeks, and hopefully longer, I challenge you to commit to at least one. Choose based on your personal needs and desires. You have your AP/AG to help. *WARNING: Not all challenges are suitable for everyone. Please see your health care provider for any questions regarding your personal challenge choices.*

1. **Water Challenge**—Drink 64 ounces of water every day (or recommended amount)
2. **Vegetable Challenge***—eat 5 servings of vegetables every day
3. **Super Vegetable Challenge***—eat 12 servings of vegetables every day
4. **Eat 3 Servings of Vegetables at Meals**—breakfast, lunch, and dinner
5. **No Yeast Challenge**—do not consume any foods with yeast
6. **Sugar Challenge**—do not eat more than 20 grams of "added sugars" per day
7. **No Processed Foods Challenge**—do not eat anything that is prepackaged
8. **Eggs & Oatmeal Breakfast Challenge**—limit options; eat healthy for breakfast
9. **No Alcohol Challenge**—do not drink any alcohol
10. **No Soda Challenge**—do not drink soda
11. **No Carbonation Challenge**—do not drink anything carbonated
12. **No Fatty Meat Challenge**—do not eat any fatty meats, or fat from the meat
13. **No Dairy Challenge**—if you suspect an intolerance, do not consume lactose
14. **No Gluten Challenge**—if you suspect an intolerance, do not eat foods containing gluten
15. **No Bread Challenge**—do not eat bread or anything that resembles it
16. **No White Food Challenge**—do not consume white creams, sauces, butter, or flour
17. **No Salt Challenge**—do not pick up that salt shaker; limit heavy sodium foods
18. **No Cookie Challenge**—do not eat any cookies
19. **No Frozen Dinner Challenge**—do not eat any prepackaged frozen dinners
20. **Eat 3 Meals Per Day Challenge**—do not skip meals
21. **Water Before Meal Challenge**—drink one large glass of water before every meal
22. **Track your Calories Challenge**—use an app to track every morsel and drink
23. **Past 8 PM Challenge**—do not eat after 8 pm
24. **No Eating Out Challenge**—cook and eat at home or a friend's house

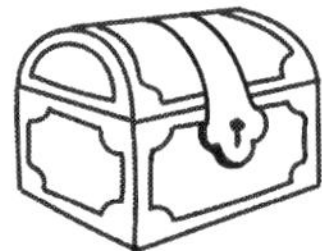

*If you need help deciding what veggies to eat, see the full list of vegetables in the Treasure Chest in the section: Meal Planning Step 4.

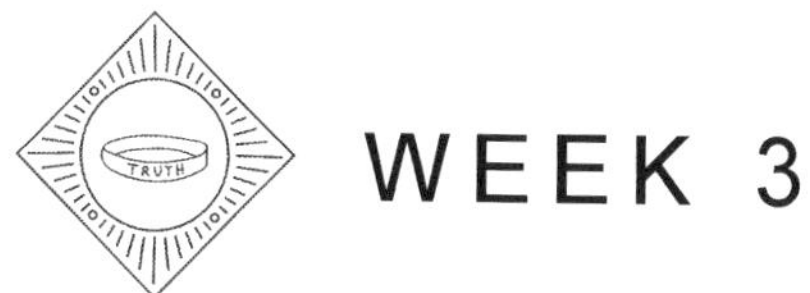

WEEK 3

ARM YOURSELF WITH TRUTH

Week 3, Day 1
Truth of the Gospel

"Stand therefore, having girded your waist with truth..."
—Ephesians 6:14a

Imagine if truth did not exist. Kids could tell lies, half truths, or embellish stories to astronomical proportions—without rebuttal. We would never really know reality from a big fat lie. But the absence of truth would not just make it impossible to distinguish a liar from a truth-teller; it would assault marriage commitments and diminish morals. This is exactly why we must follow the undeniable truth that is authentic, never upgraded, unaltered, unchanged, and constant, no matter how the emerging society tries to redefine it.

"The truth is incontrovertible. Malice may attack it, ignorance may deride it, but in the end, there it is."—Winston Churchill

Truth is in accordance with reality. Our ideas cannot change it. Our thoughts have no reflection or bearing on truth. We cannot redefine truth by deeming what God says as wrong or right. Philosophy's longest ongoing discussion is truth. I heard it said by a college student, "I don't accept all of Christ's truths because if I did, I'd have to change the way I live—and then I'd be accountable for my own eternity." This individual does not want to submit, change, or be accountable for the way they live.

The Gospel means good news. It does not mean good advice. Society has altered the definition of the Gospel by adding, subtracting, and dividing it up so that the definition fits society's ideal answer—but that does not mean the Gospel went along with it. The Gospel is still the same good news that saves us from sin and self-destruction, religion and self-righteousness. It alters the way we think, and it sets us free, makes us feel clean, and changes selfish desires supernaturally. The truth of the Gospel is not a code to follow. The truth of the Gospel is Jesus. If you truly allow His truths to penetrate your heart, He will change more than your life; He will change your eternity.

Ultimate truth is the Gospel. It is the reason and purpose for living and being. Jesus Himself is truth (John 14:6). The Gospel is truth above our own truth. It is the real truth—the forever standard, set-in-stone truth that always was, always is, and always will be. Ultimate truth will never change and is the basis of life. It is the only thing left when the world's definition of truth has vanished. It is truth that is above all others, the highest level of truth, and the standard for which to reach.

Every person has sinned (Romans 3:23). Sin separates us from God and the penalty for sin is death. Only someone who did not have sin could pay our way out of this punishment. Jesus, God's Son, was the only perfect substitute, the remedy for our brokenness, who could render this debt once and for all and cleanse us from sin. This is the only way to be rejoined with

God (read Surrender in the Treasure Chest for a better understanding). Jesus had to die for us, in our place, to rescue us from the penalty of our sins, without us helping, paying, or doing something for it. (If we had to do something to become clean, salvation would be based on works—something we did, not Jesus' sacrifice.) He paid our debt. He rose from the grave and ascended back to heaven (something no one else has matched) to show us He indeed was and is God.

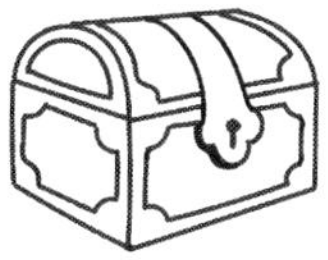

We must believe in Him in order to be with the Lord forever in heaven. This is the only way to everlasting life according to Jesus. We have to accept this truth and give our life (will, body, and emotions) to Him.

Even though the Bible was written over the course of a thousand years, it all flows and connects—from the beginning to the end. The Good News is unstoppable, it will not be snuffed out, but that does not mean it is accepted. Even Elvis Presley got it right when he said, "Truth is like the sun. You can shut it out for a time, but it ain't goin' away." We are called to gird our loins with truth, act on it, speak it, and take it everywhere we go. Believing in the truth of the Gospel of Christ is the first and most important piece of armor in this war. We need it not just to be a part of our lives, but to be the reason why we live our lives.

ARMOR ALERT: Your Ultimate Truth

1. **What do you believe is ultimate truth in your life and how do you know this *deep inside* to be true?** (My hope is that you share this answer in utmost truth with your AP/AG.)

2. **Maybe you have given Christ your life but not full control of it. Is there any area you need to surrender to Him fully?**

Week 3, Day 2
Blenders of Truth

"Stand therefore, having girded your waist with truth..."
—Ephesians 6:14a

Imagine a husband and wife who are recently married, but a few months after the vows, he drops a bomb on his bride. He says he had an affair with another woman, claims nothing really happened, and he does not want to talk about it because it is over. Would she accept this as the whole story, the whole truth, and move on? This bomb is anything but the whole truth. If he was in an affair, he did something to breach the marriage covenant. He broke his vows once, which means it could happen again—especially if there are no consequences the first time. If nothing really happened, then there was no need to admit to the affair. If it is now over, then something had to start somewhere. She would demand the full truth—all of it.

Truth is what Satan has been trying to snuff out for centuries. He spreads false truths and suggests there is more than one way to God and heaven, we need to do things to earn heaven, Jesus cannot really forgive all our secrets and sins, we need to have more faith to be healed, and hell is not a real place where good people are sent. Some religions accept Jesus as a holy prophet but nothing more. We cannot pick and choose and only believe part of what Jesus says. True prophets are never wrong (Ezek 12:25).

Giving half of the truth is deception at its greatest. We told part of the truth, so we do not feel as bad about the half we left out. Deception is Satan's specialty. His partial and half-truths are wisely blended with part of the truth so that they are accepted. The "if it sounds good it must be true" saying is usually the farthest thing from the truth. Some truth just stinks, but it does not change the truth. It does not matter how truth sounds or how it makes us feel. Our entitlement issues cannot change truth, nor can we will something to morph into truth. When we are not continually renewing our minds in the truths of the Gospel and connecting with Jesus, we slowly believe these "too good to be true" partial-truths and adopt them as our own.

At a backyard BBQ, politics, religious stabs, and false truths are thrown around like horseshoes. The Good News is reduced to good advice when it gets tossed around too much. It makes us feel like we can take it or leave it. Religious perspectives turn into differences of opinions, which could very well be why hostility is present when talking religion—it is too important to some and not important enough to others. Besides, religion can be hostile, annoying, confusing, and lead to riots, fights, and anger. The truth of the Gospel is not religious (it is not what we do or how we perform traditions or cultural ceremonies), it is grace.

If a book about the ancient Roman Empire was written last week, most would believe it, even though the author did not live during that time. There is no one to disprove the written text. The writers of the Bible, however, used first and last names to account for the facts. These people were still alive and able to refute if the facts were false, but no one did.

The Bible has many ancient artifacts to back up its claims too. More than that, it has roughly 40 different authors. It was written over the course of 1,500 years, and in that time, none of the text was ever denied or attributed as a false claim by the society in which it was written. The reason why people refute the Bible now is because if they actually believed it to be true, they would be accountable to it. The Bible becomes extremely personal, whereas other accounts of factual history do not. In our current day, we only need two witnesses to prove someone innocent or guilty in court and to distinguish truth from a lie. There were way more than two witnesses attesting Jesus was dead and then suddenly alive.

We must be on our guard against the mixers of half-truths. The number one half-truth I hear is that good people go to heaven. We are called to be good, that is indeed true, but we do not earn the right to walk through heaven's gates because of our kind acts. It is by grace that we are saved, not by our works (Ephesians 2:8-9; Titus 3:5; James 2:26). God made heaven for those who love and honor Him, not for those who want to life in a peaceful eternity so they give to the church. What baffles me is why someone who does not love Jesus, or wants to spend any time with Him now would want to spend eternity with Him. It is His eternal home that He owns and governs. It would be like me walking up to a beautiful home on earth, ringing the doorbell and telling the owners I earned the right to live with them because I am a good person and volunteer.

Another mixture of truth is that hell is not as bad as Jesus makes it out to be. The Old Testament reports hell as a real place, and Jesus' own words in the New Testament are very descriptive. In fact, He talked a lot about hell with many warnings. Satan's hell and God's heaven do exist, but they are complete opposites of each other. Heaven beholds the attributes of God, and since God is not in hell, His attributes would be the farthest thing from hell. That means in hell there is no water, strength, rest, justice, truth, health, life, hope, beauty, order, law, and definitely no love—ever. And, these are just some of God's attributes that would be missing from hell.

Satan concocted the greatest lie of all, misrepresenting hell as being a party with endless luxuries. The truth is, all you will find in this fiery pit is the opposite of God—confusion, no rights, no name, no reference as to who you once were, no hope of getting out, all the while being in the most agonizing hellish state you could not even think of in the middle of the worst nightmare possible—without escape. (Psalm 69:28; Luke 16:24-25; Revelation 14:11, 10:20)

The torments of hell will be spiritual (2 Thessalonians 1:5-9), mental and physical (Luke 16:22-25; Jude 12-13; Revelation 14:11), and emotional (Luke 16:19-31). The torture would attack our entire being from all areas—inside out.

ARMOR ALERT: Half Truths

God will not make you follow Him any more than He will make you eat healthy and exercise. Likewise, the enemy will not make us sin—that is all up to us. Eve diminished God's Word and added to it. She changed what God said to fulfill her selfish desires—the "I." It appears Adam passively went along with Eve. Society can easily persuade us to go along quietly with their definitions of truth too. We are all free to choose, but not free to choose our consequences.

1. **Do you believe you are going to heaven? If so, do you know of any Scriptures for your defense or any reasons why?**

2. **Write some comments from these past two days that concerned you, warned you, enlightened you, or that you need more clarity about. Discuss these with your AP.**

Week 3, Day 3
Don't Take the Bait

"And Jesus said to them, 'I am the bread of life. He who comes to Me shall never hunger, and he who believes in Me shall never thirst.'"
—John 6:35

As I laid on the gurney being prepped to deliver twin girls, I was having second thoughts, even though this was my fifth delivery in six years. You see, in my previous deliveries, I had an excellent help agent called an epidural, which allowed me to push through those intense portions of labor without the screaming I was currently hearing down the hall. This time around, however, I faced the incomparable news that it was too late for such help.

I doubted my abilities because I knew this time I would be forced to meet pain head on—and possibly a double portion of it. I realized millions of other women labored this path before and made it to the other side, so I was confident I would too. It is just entirely different when we foresee the pain, and there is no way of getting out. I realized I did not know the depths of my abilities to deliver these sweet babies until I was challenged beyond my known capabilities. (*We are done having kids by the way. Some challenges don't need to be repeated.*) All this being said, my own pain seems so insignificantly minuscule compared to what Jesus went through in those hours before He was nailed to the cross.

"I realized I did not know the depths of my abilities to deliver these sweet babies until I was challenged beyond my known capabilities."

Jesus knew He was going to face not only physical pain but also separation from God. None of us can comprehend the agony and mind-blowing path that was set before Him, but He knew exactly who He was and why He was headed to the cross. When I listen to the "I," it is easy to be confused on who I really am—and where I am headed. I question if God is calling me to take this step or that one, go in this direction or not. *"I" am not good enough. "I" am not strong enough. "I" can't do that, God!* I feel like a flag wafting in the winds of doubt. Jesus never wavered.

Doubt is like water. When we listen to it, even for a second, it seeps in and begins to fill our hearts. The absolute best way to arm ourselves, and drown out doubt, is to use Scripture. These sacred words written long ago are actually living and active. This is why we hear people call the Bible the "Living Word of God." Use the Scriptures found in the Treasure Chest, Scriptures to Combat Doubt & Fear, to deflate the enemy's attacks instead of using paper swords and attempting to be positive, trying yet another medication, or *willing* a way to freedom. God's Word is stronger than a two-edged sword. This means Scripture can turn off doubt. Declare these

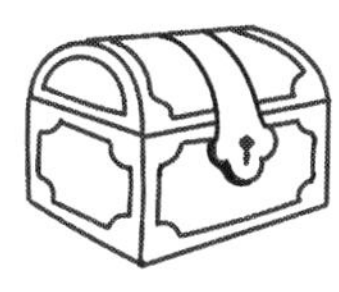

truths from the Bible over your life, will, and health by reading and renewing your mind with God's Word whenever doubt comes looking for a fight.

By now you are getting more glimpses of how this spiritual battle relates to your overall health, but what if I were to tell you that nutrition fallouts are more spiritual in nature than we physically claim them to be? These evil forces do not make us eat poorly or be lazy. They do not make us do anything—that is all on us. However, they suggest and throw those ideas out there like bait dangling from a shiny line (since women like shiny things—it tempts us). When we are aware of the sly enemy's plan and arm ourselves with an effective spiritual plan, we have a better shot at controlling our nutritional habits.

I never realized the bait luring me in until I prayed and asked God why I kept going back to my weekend overeating. I would eat super well during the week but let loose and consume everything in sight over the weekend. I knew I was a repeat offender, even though I would try to stop. I would feel so proud of myself when I would stay on the straight and narrow all week, but somewhere along the line, I got this feeling that I could reward myself and eat whatever I wanted at the end of the week. I was taking the bait. This stumbling block was forged in my mind—planted there somehow, by someone, or by something. How could it be that my very goal of trying to lose weight by consuming less was rewarded by eating terrible on my days off? This obvious failure made me feel embarrassed, shameful, and upset at myself.

I began to doubt if I would ever trust myself to do it right. Once I realized what game was being played, I decided to shut down the "free weekend eating" and make healthy eating a lifestyle. Sure I could have treats here and there, but those were the key words—here and there. Doubts will come, and challenges will always be before us, both big and small, with ourselves and with other areas in life. One thing we should always strive for is to be secure in our faith by connecting with God on a deeper level. The more we honestly connect with God, the more we will hear His voice, and the less we will listen to the "I" of doubt and the bait of the enemy.

Focus on the highlights. If you feel accomplished about hitting a health goal, savor the moment and think about how you can make that moment last longer. Reward yourself with a positive approach. If restricting food, do not reward yourself with food. Choose something else like a movie, date night, or a trip, purchase memorabilia, write about it, etc.

ARMOR ALERT: Stop Doubting & Start Yearning

We are told to love God with all our heart, soul, mind, and strength (Mark 12:28-29), and that we will be blessed and satisfied because of it. "Blessed are those who hunger and thirst for righteousness, for they will be filled" (Matthew 5:6). "Jesus is the bread of life," means He sustains us physically and spiritually. We should hunger and thirst (yearn, desire, long) for

Christ as we do food (sugar, fried foods, carbs, chocolate) and water (soda, alcohol, coffee). He gives us nourishment that is spiritual and sustaining forever.

1. **Why do people sometimes love food more than God?**

2. **If you want to thirst and desire God more than food, it starts by spending time with Him. Take time today and tell Him all about it.**

Trainer Talk

How's your 2-Week Nutrition Challenge going? What about your exercise? Adding these two elements together is a recipe for physical health. I've prayed for you to succeed in these areas. Ask God to give you strength and discipline—He will help when you go to Him. You got this!

Week 3, Day 4
Who's Leading Whom?

"Do not be wise in your own eyes; fear the LORD and depart from evil.
It will be health to your flesh, and strength to your bones."
—Proverbs 3:7-8

One night as I tucked my six-year-old in bed, she asked why they don't let Jesus be the line leader at school. My simple answer was that some kids don't believe in Jesus. But once I thought a little longer, I realized it is truly because most of us want to be the leader instead. That's when it hit me. I immediately knew I was not letting Jesus be the line leader in my life all the time. I was allowing the "I" to lead instead. When it comes down to it, if we obeyed and listened to all the truths in the Bible, our lives would change. We would not want to be the leader anymore and would unwaveringly love Jesus so much; we would completely trust Him to lead us one hundred percent of the time.

If people think they have a good life, why would they need to change anything? After all, if they do not seemingly have any problems, they wouldn't need to bring God into it. However, as soon as a disease, loss of a loved one, or a job becomes too big for their command, God is summoned immediately. We all intuitively know we need Him, we just do not want Him to disrupt the "I" too much. God gives us abundant joy and health to our bones, but not when we follow the "I."

The Bible tells us many things about our health, and one thing is for sure—His truths can make us healthy. We shouldn't be wise in our own eyes (relying on the "I") We should fear the LORD, and depart from evil (Satan's rebellion of selfishness). The Bible says it will be health to our navel, and marrow to thy bones (Proverbs 3:7-8). Health does not mean physically healthy alone. According to this verse, when we give God full reign of our minds (listening to God instead of the "I") and hand off any false claims on truth (the half-truths of the enemy), our bones can be healthy. Think spiritually with me. When our soul is rotten, it affects us spiritually. Sin is like cancer to our soul. It makes us rotten from the inside out, spreading and trying to ruin everything good in its path. Cancer of the soul is more devastating than the physical counterpart. Our present physical condition will pale in comparison to our eternal spiritual state if separated from God.

We do not know all the complex intricacies of the spirit world. We are only given glimpses, but we do know it tries to bait and destroy us in every area of our health. "A sound heart is the life of the flesh: but envy the rottenness to the bones" (Proverbs 14:30). God's Word is saying that when we are not at peace with Him, these spiritually-rooted diseases of the heart (such as envy) can manifest themselves physically (rottenness of our bones). These invisible diseases can make us mentally stressed, emotionally compromised, and physically ill. This means the spiritual world crosses into the physical—which is honestly hard to wrap our minds around. We know deep inside this exchange takes place, but the mysterious invisible realm is truly a mystery of sorts. When we make the "I" leader, the enemy comes in and takes an assignment of destruction (John 10:10). If we make Jesus the leader, He promises we can be healthy in our innermost being.

You can do more *with* God than without Him. Look all through the HIStory (HIS Story—God's story) of the Bible. You will find actual history on how people overcame battles no matter the condition of their flesh because they allowed God to lead. When God's people allowed Him to be their line leader, they won physical battles in supernatural ways (the Bible refers to battles over 185 times). Moses gave God the lead to part the Red Sea so His chosen people could physically cross on dry ground. Moses and the Israelites did not do their part on their own strength—God did it supernaturally. Samson did not muster enough physical strength to collapse a building with his bare hands while chained (killing more enemies at once than in the sum of his lifetime) all by his physical self. God gave him supernatural strength when he surrendered fully to the Lord. Apart from God, we can do nothing (John 15:5b).

Jesus had constant communication with the Father and never allowed the "I" to be the leader. He stayed on the straight and narrow. This is how Jesus so amazingly fulfilled His earthly ministry to the very end when on the cross He released the words, "It is finished." Jesus can supernaturally help you win battles if you allow Him to lead your life.

ARMOR ALERT: Who is Your Line Leader?

Today isn't loaded with a lot of questions to answer. First, take some time to ponder your relationship with God. Then, record any area in your life where Jesus is not the line leader.

Trainer Talk

Be mindful that life happens and setbacks with exercise or nutrition are very normal—even in the middle of a health program. This allows us to reach out to God and ask Him for strength, instead of being proud of our strong will. Give Jesus credit for any accomplishments and continue to ask Him to help you throughout the challenges that are coming. How many times have you worked out this week? Are you sticking to your plan?

Before You Meet

Put on the Belt of Truth

Moment for Meditation

Lord God,

You are amazing and powerful. Thank You for being a holy and just God. Thank You for giving me the truth. Help me put the belt of truth around my waist every day. Help me recognize Your truths, and not to go left or right, but to stay on your path. Give me wisdom to stand up for Your truths, regardless what the current society dictates.

Show me when truth is not present and keep my eyes open to recognize the false ones. Be my guide and help me not to take the bait of doubt. I want to follow You at all times.

Lord, please forgive me of any offenses and cleanse me. Keep truth on my lips, guarded around my waist, and in my heart. I give You my all.

Thank You. Amen.

IT'S TIME TO MEET!

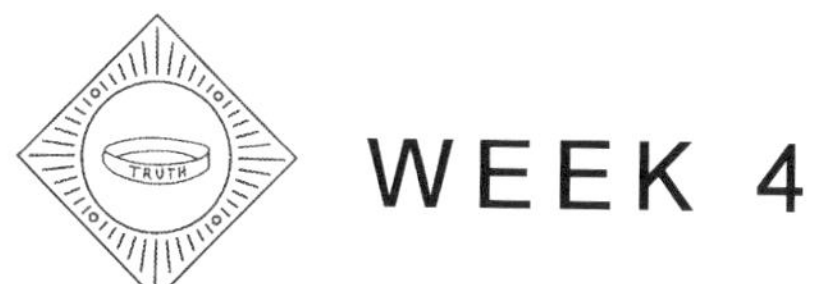

WEEK 4

ARM YOURSELF WITH NUTRITIONAL HEALTH

Week 4, Day 1
Banking on Your Health

"Wisdom is the principal thing; therefore get wisdom.
And in all your getting, get understanding."
—Proverbs 4:7

Imagine a bank account that was opened in your name when you were born. Your parents diligently deposited a monthly sum and once a high school graduate, your parents gifted you the generous amount. This investment required diligence, patience, and sacrifice—and took planning. This is exactly how we must approach the gift of our health. We cannot bank on our health without making nutritional deposits. I am going to warn you, this week will take some planning, patience, and sacrifice as well, and likewise, it will have a huge payoff in the end. If you are too busy to carve out time to evaluate your nutrition this week, ask God to multiply your time. Now, let's get a little education under our "belts" and learn why we need nutrition so desperately.

If we purchased a new sports car, we would not come home and put junky oil or watered down gasoline in it. Have you ever wondered why we allow the worst nutritional fuels to go down our tanks? Our material possessions seem to have a better investment plan than our physical bodies. Once we are educated and realize the importance of healthy food, we will have a harder time investing in the wrong things and filling up with poor choices.

What current deposits are you making with your nutrition?

We make time for what we truly desire. I have to focus and make time to eat healthy. It is a sacrifice, just like when we invest monetarily into our bank accounts. A little bit of time pays off in the end. If we eat healthy for two weeks straight, we will naturally feel better, but then we cannot just call it quits and go back to old habits and expect that small investment to sustain us for any length of time. Eating healthy has dividends in the future—sometimes farther than we think. If I fail to plan with food, my family ends up eating on the go, and we pay for it later (my kids don't feel good, they get cranky, and don't sleep well either). It does take time to plan and prepare healthy food, just as it takes time to lose weight with exercise, but that time invested pays off in the end.

When I feed my kids crackers, they can polish off three to four times the suggested serving size. The generic cracker serving size is about five pieces, but the average kid never wants just five crackers—they want a lot more. When we eat an apple, we are satisfied and usually do not want another apple. It is so the opposite with our favorite cookie, as I am one to suggest just give me the box. I do not need another, "I" want another.

When we make poorly packaged food choices, more of those foods are required to fill us up. These are usually simple carbohydrates (sugary snacks, bleached white flour muffins, crackers, chips, etc.), which do not make us feel full for any length of time. Vegetables are more complex and have vitamins and minerals (micronutrients) as well as complex carbohydrates (a macronutrient) that take longer to break down in our tummies. We need to eat fewer veggies to fill up, and they fuel us longer than a handful of crackers. I know vegetables are not near as exciting to eat as packaged foods, but give them a chance. Your desires just might not be established yet.

Ladies, if you are raising a family or have a spouse to cook for, BE THE BEST YOU CAN BE in this area for them! If you have growing children in your home, think about their bodies, bones, cells, and muscles that are forming the very building blocks of their adult frames. Simple planning can save your wallet and your waistline because it takes more money to make us unhealthy (going out to eat costs more).

An easy way to make my kids eat well is to buy only healthy foods. When there is no junk food around, and they revolt with a refusal plan, they will eventually get hungry and eat what is there. I do buy some junk foods, but once these are gone, I do not buy more. I cannot allow my children to make all of their diet choices. We need to help teach them not to be controlled by the "I" right alongside us—and this is possibly true about our spouses, too. We all know food choices will not be the only thing the "I" will try to control. Our kids will venture out and try the "I" in other areas. I want my husband to be around after our children have grown. He might not like the new meal plan either, but marriage is for better or worse. Tell him if he thinks this is the worst part, he can get the better later.

ARMOR ALERT: Meal Planning

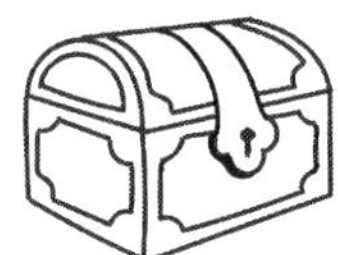

In the Treasure Chest, go to Meal Planning Step 1: Identify Your Real Consumption. Your goal is to either continue with the meal plan you are using or go through this simple program and create your very own. This could be overwhelming if you don' thave the time to do this. Set time aside to concentrate. This is such an important part of your health and could change your life. Do not feel like you have to do all of Step 1 in a day or even in a week. Use it as a tool now to push the start button and come back to it in the future if needed.

Take the time to ponder what you read and don't skip ahead. Step 2 is coming up soon enough.

Trainer Talk

You may have learned a lot of new information so far, but there is more left to swallow. If you aren't moving through your 2-Week Challenge with momentum, don't worry. This is a challenge, and challenges are supposed to be hard. Utilize your AP. If time is an issue and you forget to eat, set an alarm on your phone to remind you. Remember to keep moving forward in your daily exercise—stick to your plan. If your plan isn't working, change it and try something different.

Week 4, Day 2
The Master Nutritionist

"So, whether you eat or drink, or whatever you do, do all to the glory of God."
—2 Corinthians 10:31

Thousands of nutritional advice books cover bookstore shelves and the web. It is a hot topic and for good reason—we are massively unhealthy and need intervention. With too many suggestions of how, what, and when to eat, the amount of advice can be overwhelming. Searching for the latest way science declares the new nutritional standard can make anyone exhausted. This is why we should trust the One who made our food supply and the bodies we use to consume it. God gave us His favorite seafood options and told us not to be drunk or eat raw meat. He says never to drink blood and gives His preferred animals and insects to consume. He even instructs us to eat honey minimally. God reveals His food standards in the Bible, as the Master Nutritionist.

Leviticus and Deuteronomy are filled with food requirements from God, along with the consequences for the Israelites if they did not obey. Many people ask if Old Testament food laws are for us today. The controversial and part answer is yes. This is not to say if we eat from the "do not eat" list we will be defiled spiritually. In the opening paragraphs of Genesis, God clearly gave us plants to eat. After the flood, God told Noah in Genesis 9:3 that every moving and living thing was food for them. We can eat anything, but it does not mean it is good longevity food. Processed food is edible, we can eat it, but that does not mean it will provide a stable nutritious living. We can eat drive-thru food often, but be we'll reap the consequences. Let's say I have a personal conviction to not eat pork, but someone else may farm pigs and have no conviction at all about eating these animals. God could be calling us to various convictions at different times—we just need to be obedient whenever His prompting comes.

"Let thy food be thy medicine and thy medicine be thy food."— Hippocrates (460-377 B.C.)

God commanded food requirements in the Old Testament for His reasons, the most obvious is learning to be obedient. Since God is *all-knowing* and created our bodies, there may be a few reasons beyond obedience. Consider the possibility that God established laws for sanitary reasons and the general health of His people. In Leviticus 11, God had to separate the Israelites from other nations with what we think as some unusual laws. However, they are not illogical. They are packed with deeper meaning, some of which we might never fully understand.

The laws for that period, such as abstaining from unnatural sexual relationships and killing everyone in an evil city, were also for physical protection. Laws protected back then, and they still do today. Even though most of us eat foods from His unclean list, there are still basic natural consequences if we consume in large quantities. In short, poor food choices still harm our bodies and promote side effects.

God commanded His chosen never to drink blood, as recorded in Leviticus 3:17. They were to drain the blood and cook the meat instead of eating it raw. Before there were mechanized agricultural equipment and refrigeration, there were visible spoiling and contamination issues. Not only were there limitations on how long something could be kept out in hot weather, but also there were safe food handling and raw meat consumption instructions that did not exactly make the front page of the *Old Testament Times*. We now have science to prove blood-borne pathogens are present in raw meats that can make our physical bodies very sick and can even cause death.

God told His chosen not to eat certain sea creatures. Sure they may taste good when covered with butter (almost anything does), but think about what these creatures eat. Some of them are bottom dwellers and eat from the sea floor. They clean up waste from other creatures. There is a reason why God said this is not the best choice for our bodies. We now have scientific proof that shows high mercury levels are fatal to humans, levels which are found in some of these unapproved creatures. God had known this before science confirmed it. He told us long ago in the Bible as The Master Nutritionist.

If you have read about Daniel in the Bible, you might remember when King Nebuchadnezzar took the Jews captive to Babylon. He decided to take the good men and keep them for service in his courts. For them to appear strong and serve him, they had to be trained for three full years. During this time of strict training, the trainees had to eat the king's delectable choice foods and wine. Daniel appealed to the chief guard on account of the Law. He asked if he and his buddies could eat only veggies and water for 10 days as a trial. After that, the guards could compare their physical state with those who ate the king's royal diet. The guard reluctantly agreed. After 10 days, the chief guard was shocked at how strong and healthy Daniel and his friends appeared. They were even much farther ahead with their abilities to think and process information. It was such a difference that the chief guard changed the regulations so that everyone had to eat like Daniel did for training to serve the king.

If hundreds of years ago a revelation as simple as eating vegetables and water for 10 days proved these men could rise above all others, why wouldn't we consider this way of eating for ourselves—just for 10 days? We know very well the reason we do not run to these opportunities with joy. The "I" is getting in the way, isn't it? Cutting our contemporary comforts and conveniences for this kind of diet does not sound appealing, even for two days.

Many authors have penned books about Daniel's way of eating to highlight the importance of this ancient Biblical diet. It is a super clean way to eat, and is simple, because it takes so much stress out of the equation with little time needed to prepare food. Consider trying a commitment to this diet for 10 days to see how different you feel.

Sometimes when we go through a new way of eating, it can make our mental, physical and emotional states uneasy. Be prepared—if you restrict your body of these comforts, it usually revolts big time. I will be totally honest—I was nervous when I first thought of going *plant only* for 10 days. I thought I would miss protein and fats and not be able to consume enough calories, but plants have everything we need for survival, and you get to eat a lot. This diet was a divinely appointed way of eating by God to enhance the human body, inside out.

ARMOR ALERT: Go-To List

1. **Make a list of five go-to items you keep on hand that is healthy in the space to the right of my lists. These should not be anything dramatic that you have to think about or make. As you can see my examples below, I like to include salty, sweet, hearty, crunchy, and hot and spicy options in my list. Use your list when you have no idea what to eat but need something quick. You can change them seasonally or change them monthly.**

   Sarah's Go-To List—Fall & Winter
   1. Flat Pretzels—Salty
   2. Apples—Sweet
   3. Organic Granola Cereal—Crunchy
   4. Hard Boiled Egg—Hearty
   5. Celery & Peanut Butter—Crunchy

   Sarah's Go-To List—Weekend
   1. Air Popped Popcorn—Salty
   2. Sweet potato—Sweet
   3. Baby Carrots—Crunchy
   4. Cottage Cheese—Hearty
   5. Red Peppers and Hummus—Bitter

2. **Once you have completed your Go-To List, go to the Treasure Chest and continue with Meal Planning Step 2: Get a Grip on the Food Label.**

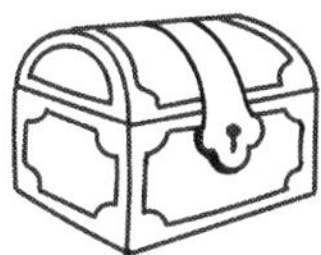

Week 4, Day 3
Truth Behind Your Calories

"Do you not know that you are the temple of God and that the Spirit of God dwells in you?"
—1 Corinthians 3:16

God is so mathematical it blows me away. He even uses math formulas in our food sources. His forethought when creating us is incredible. Foods we are not addicted to, such as cucumbers, do not make us fat. The foods we are easily addicted to, like chips, can leave us with devastating consequences. This is to ensure consequences if we are addicted to anything other than God. Sugar is obviously addictive. This sweet source is loaded with empty calories. When we over-consume, we are besieged with extra body fat—among other health issues. It only gives us momentary satisfaction, and leaves us with baggage in the end (this should remind us of sin). Eating sugar is not a sin, but being addicted to it is another story. God desires for us to have balance in our lives (Goldilocks), and to be addicted to Him alone.

I can't even fathom how incredible God is and am constantly amazed the more I study how food metabolically breaks down and converts in our bodies. Calories are the body's energy currency and are essential for daily activity. If we do not use all the calories we consume during the day, they are stored and converted elsewhere for various tasks. This impressive balance of the right amount should be the goal we aim to achieve. We should not consume too much, or consume too little. The total number of calories a person needs each day varies with a few factors including age, gender, height, weight, activities of daily living, and level of physical activity. Even if you do not exercise, you burn calories all day just by being alive and breathing. This process is called your daily caloric necessities, or your BMR (Basal Metabolic Rate).[2]

3,500 calories equal one pound. The average woman needs about 1,800-2,200 calories per day depending on activity level according to the FDA.[3] If you currently consume 1,800 calories per day and want to lose weight, you have three natural options:

1. Reduce your calories.
2. Increase your exercise to burn more calories.
3. Combine both numbers 1 and 2.

In order to lose weight, it helps if you know how many calories you are currently eating. Thanks to the FDA, they require printed calorie counts on the back of all food labels. Food labels show a general 2,000 calorie diet. You can experiment with your calorie intake and activity level to find a good fit for you. *Regardless of your desires, never consume less than 1,200 calories per day unless directed by a physician. If you have concerns with your caloric intake, please make an appointment with a local health professional.

Tracking food and calories makes us aware of what we place in our mouths. A few handfuls of food in the evening could mean the difference between gaining or losing weight. You can track your calories electronically (myfoodpyramind.gov or myfitnesspal.com). If you choose these free websites/apps, they add up your calories as well as vitamins, minerals, carbs, fats, sugars, and more for you. You can also share your food log with your AP/AG.

"My people are destroyed from lack of knowledge..." (Hosea 4:6). Just because you stay under your calorie goal does not mean you are healthy. If you consumed only vegetables and water for 10 days, like Daniel, and I gobbled up only drive-thru food, and we both ate a 2,000 calorie diet, who do you think would be healthier? You consumed whole foods that metabolized more efficiently and aided in rebuilding muscles—far superior to the drive-thru food. Since you did not eat as many junky calories, you would be healthier, just like Daniel and his buddies.

A banana is about 70 calories and a cookie about 140 calories. It costs less to eat a banana than to gobble up a cookie—plus, we do not just eat one cookie. It is also cheaper to get rid of the calories from one banana than from four cookies. It costs us far less to eat healthy than to eat more and gain weight.

We must have balance in our food with carbs, proteins, and fats. If we only ate carbohydrates, which is our energy source, and no protein to rebuild muscles, we would turn into a blob of blubber. If we only ate protein and not fat, we would shrivel up and be a mental mess as our brains would lack the fat needed to function. Balance is one of the most important challenges we can run after.

ARMOR ALERT: Spreading Them Out

Many skip breakfast, power through lunch with a wimpy 200-calorie salad, and then by dinner they are starving. Friends, if you eat this way, you *should be* starving. You just starved yourself most of the day and were not fueled during the most crucial hours. The afternoon or late evening is when most overeat and gorge, binge eat, and consume poor choices to compensate.

1. **Go to the Treasure Chest, Meal Planning Step 3: Identify Your Caloric Goals. Once you complete this step, go to question number two below.**

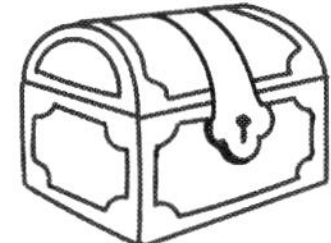

2. **Use this chart below to help figure out the best option for you. Circle the closest calorie option below and plug this into your daily tracking application. The goal is to spread calories out—so you are not consuming most of them at dinner.**

Breakfast	Snack	Lunch	Snack	Dinner	Snack	Total
400	200	600	100	600	100	2000
400	100	500	100	600	100	1800
400	100	500	100	500	100	1700
400	100	500	100	400	100	1600
400	100	400	100	400	100	1500
400		400	100	400	100	1400
400		400	100	400		1300
400		400		400		1200

Week 4, Day 4
What To Eat?

"The plans of the diligent lead surely to plenty, but those of everyone who is hasty, surely to poverty."
—Proverbs 21:5

It's now 5 PM and I have nothing for dinner! No plans, no meat, no time, and no desire. The out-to-eat meal plans are beginning to form. I have been in this position so many times. Regardless of what tools you learn in these next few weeks, this scenario will most likely happen to you too, but the frequency of it is what you will learn to decrease.

I eat similar things all week long. When I buy fresh blueberries, it is easier to eat them during those seven days instead of freezing and thawing them for the following week. After I eat blueberries the first week, I am ready for a different type of berry. If I buy extra eggs one week, I can boil the ones I do not eat right away and enjoy them in a different way the following week. Schedules can change often enough, but my foods do not have to until my family and I become bored with them. Dinner usually costs the most and is often the highest pressure-filled meal. Since we all eat the same breakfast and lunch choices daily, by dinner, we want something different and without repeats.

Many Americans do not seem to consume enough vitamins and minerals from natural food choices, so they pop in a pill. This can be very helpful, but the favored option is to get these from your foods first. God made your nutrients packaged and ready to consume in the form of fresh fruits and veggies. Fresh fruit even has a disposable wrapper—the peel. They are fabulous snacks or complements to any meal. Fruit has fiber, which makes us feel fuller longer. Fiber is essential to move things in our systems. Fiber is one of the first things I look at when buying a protein bar. If it has less than five grams of fiber, it doesn't go in my basket.

Since vitamins are essential for our health, and most of us aren't getting enough from our foods, how do we know if we are getting enough? This is why it is so important to track our food intake. This week you will have the opportunity to create your own meal plan from foods that you will eat—and learn how to track your daily intake. However, even if you have a plan, it needs to be accessible and habit-forming so you continue with it once these few weeks together is over.

We tend to grab what is easy and fast out of habit. I tell my clients often, "Change your meal prep habits, and you can change your health quickly." One of the easiest ways to control your nutrition is to make food preparation easy. If food prep is simple, chances are you will stick to the plan. To limit my trips to the grocery store, I spend roughly 15 minutes planning dinner, lunch, snack, and breakfast meals for a 2-week span before I go to the store. Here are just a few simple ideas to try this week.

- Take 5 minutes and cut up a whole bunch of veggies
- Buy precut veggies from the grocery store
- If you can't consume the larger container of bought veggies before they go bad, toss them in a salad or juicer, place them in veggie soup, beef stew, stir-fry, or pot pie
- Keep fruit on the counter so you can grab that instead of a packaged option
- Cook double meat and save half for tomorrow
- Make two lasagnas instead of one—freeze the other one

Even if we eat whole foods, we can still overeat and gain weight. Portion control is hard to spot. Two main tips that are easy to remember that can help when sitting down for a meal. First, all the food on our plates should not be larger than one of our outstretched hands. Second, it can take up to 20 minutes for our stomachs to transmit the message to our brains that we are indeed full. Focus on eating slowly. This will give you more time to enjoy your meal with the company you love.

I hear the statement often, "I'm cutting out all fats because that's how I lose weight." If you cut out all your fat, you are doing your body a huge disservice. When people cut out their fats, they cut out junk food, which *will* make them lose weight. However, do not be fleeced by weight loss claims to eat non-fat foods only. We have to consume healthy fats to function. A healthy range of daily fat intake is 20%-35% of our total daily intake of food, according to the FDA.[4] This can throw clients off a little, as most think it is too high. This is because the media has taught our minds that no fat is a good thing. It is all a ploy to purchase low-fat items, which are not always the best choice. We cannot afford to limit good fats because they help increase brain function, lower cholesterol, and build overall healthy cells. Limit table sugar if you are going to restrict something because it packs on the pounds—and very quickly.

God calls us to be prepared, have balance, and set goals. When we do not plan healthy meals, we usually find a poor substitute. In order to make smart choices with our meal planning, we need to know what is hiding in our foods. If you consume foods that are not packaged, you will know exactly what is in them. To improve the texture, shelf life, and flavor stability of foods, food manufacturers use partially hydrogenated oils. About half of the trans fat we consume is formed during food processing, and partially hydrogenated oils are the main source of this type of trans fat in the United States. The FDA does not require foods with less than .5 grams of trans fat to record that information on the outside of the package.[5] Since we are large-portion consumers, and consume more than the recommended amount, we could unknowingly take in over 1 gram of trans fat.

If we were trying to lose weight, we would not want to use up our daily carbohydrate intake on a few cups of fiber-less macaroni and cheese. We could eat more food with better residuals if we chose something else, like vegetables, wild rice, quinoa, or a bowl of oatmeal.

The amount of protein we should consume is calculated with our body weight. If math is not your thing to pair with nutrition, protein intake should be a percentage of your suggested daily caloric intake—pending your activity level. Not everyone should consume the same amount of protein. As a society, we are huge carnivores and being pushed to consume protein powders, specialty yogurts, and protein-enriched packaged foods and bars—more than we should. It seems we could be getting too much and not the right kinds because they are loaded with other questionable ingredients.

ARMOR ALERT: Creating a Meal Plan

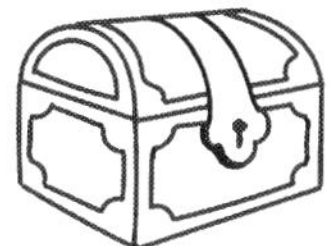

This is an exciting section loaded with ideas on how to help you achieve at your meal planning.

1. **Go to Meal Planning Step 4: Choosing Wisely, and try to finish this fun section in one sitting.**

2. **Continue with Meal Planning Step 5: Putting It Together—Simply.** (This is your chance to put it all together and pick the things you want to include in your meal plan.)

Testimony

My biggest challenge has been eating healthy. Outwardly, it wouldn't appear to be the issue, because I don't appear overweight. However, my choices weren't always the best. In fact, they were terrible, leading to lots of guilt and frustration with myself. I knew the right choices and the right foods to eat; they were right in front of me, but it was always a battle of self-will. I would choose the cookies over the apple or a handful of chips instead of veggies. Really, it just tasted better, but it was always followed by self-condemnation.

The battle in my mind was with failure. *Why can't I overcome this area?* It wasn't until this study that I realized there was more to my struggles with my eating habits. I needed to put on the Armor of God in all areas of my life.

By addressing several key areas within the study, I was able to present them to God and ask for His help and strength to make positive changes. The amount of information available for healthy eating can be overwhelming, but I found the resources for healthy snacks and meals to be a great and easy way to get back on track to eating healthy!

Tammy Bullock
Park View, IA

Before You Meet

Revisit your Pre-Evaluation Chart for a moment. How do you feel these past two weeks have helped with your nutrition? Are any actions on the left side of the chart getting closer to the right side?

Left side of chart: unscheduled, a meal-skipper, addicted, unplanned, apathetic, unhealthy, a binge eater, uncontrolled, gluttonous, obese, uneducated, craving

Right side of chart: scheduled, controlled, healthy, aware, confident, not addicted, committed, sustainable, planned, educated, not craving

Trainer Talk

Hey Beautiful, I am very proud of you for sticking with this longer nutrition portion. For some, this is a fun activity, and for others, it may seem like dreadful homework. This is the longest week and had the most written activity sandwiched in it. These essential tools will help arm you for future battles concerning food choices. I am confident you can retain this information if you participated in the previous pages. Be amazing today in your nutritional choices. If you feel like you fail in your plan, shake it off and get back into the next day. Ask God to help you be even better at it tomorrow.

Think about your 2-Week Challenge. Give yourself an overall rating of 1 out of 10 (10 being 100 percent healthy). Your goal is to treat your nutrition as a life style. Choose healthy options that are sustainable for you personally. Don't look on the goals of others if that is something you aren't ready to do. Focus on your personal goals. It will bring you much more enjoyment and fulfillment.

Do not forget to put on your belt of truth daily in the weeks ahead. Remember—in everything you do, do it all for God's glory!

When you meet next with your AP, look her in the eyes and tell her what you like about one of her habits, or characteristics.

IT'S TIME TO MEET!

SECTION THREE

BREASTPLATE OF RIGHTEOUSNESS

Your journey continues by adding another piece of the Armor of God—the breastplate of righteousness. This is our focus for the first week of this section. The second week covers the corresponding component of armor that affects our emotional health.

A breastplate covers our heart, just as righteousness can lead it. Mark 7:20 tells us that evil things like sexual immorality, murder, adultery, coveting, deceit, and more will defile us, and all comes from our heart. It is imperative that we take care of our heart and be intentional about protecting it, because letting it follow the "I" could cost us more than we want to pay.

Now, let's start off to a fabulous week by diving in a new challenge, the 2-Week Emotional Challenge.

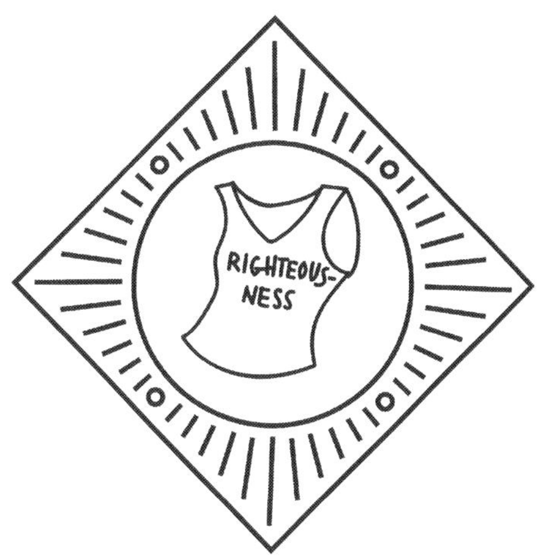

Week 5: Arm Yourself with Righteousness
Week 6: Arm Yourself with Emotional Health

Health Challenge #2
2-Week Emotional Challenge

This challenge is very personal because it is particular to you. Due to our uniqueness, we are tested differently. Emotional challenges are compelling because they flex and strengthen the muscle that encourages us to act with integrity.

Choose something deep down you need to focus on.

1. Completely unplug from technology, social media, games on your phone, or whatever vice is holding you hostage and robbing your time.
2. Find rest in your day by either taking a 15-minute power nap or getting a restful 7 to 8 hours of sleep.
3. Be intentional about spending time with someone who needs it.
4. Get artsy with paint, create music, write poetry, or make pottery.
5. Mandate one full rest day every week for your body, mind, and heart by just enjoying God and relationships—think Sabbath.
6. Sign up to be in a skit, play, or musical, or watch one.
7. Create a journal and write down every time you saw God momentsin your life.
8. Create a journal for you and your family to write encouraging notes back and forth.
9. Make a list of everything you are grateful for and then post it where you can see it every day.
10. Speak to your friend/family member about a matter you have been putting off.
11. Compliment someone you are jealous of and pray for them every day.
12. Ask God if He is calling you to be mentored by someone, then pray for who that mentor should be.
13. Evaluate your character with a list of pros and cons, and pray over it.
14. Ask God to show you how to depart from negative friendships, and follow through with it.
15. Only listen to inspirational music.
16. Look at yourself in the mirror and tell yourself one different compliment each day.
17. If your heart is bitter or hardened toward someone, seek ways to show love to that person.
18. Pray and practice self-control if you scream, shout, or yell your frustrations.
19. Read a book outside of your normal patterns and perspectives.
20. If something bad happens, do not run to a friend first—run to God.

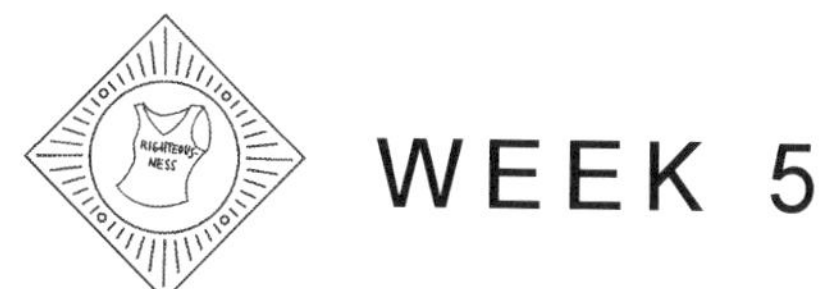

WEEK 5

ARM YOURSELF WITH RIGHTEOUSNESS

Week 5, Day 1
Righteousness

"Stand therefore, having girded your waist with truth, having put on the breastplate of righteousness…"
—Ephesians 6:14

Without a breastplate in battle, a warrior would be quickly taken out with his vital organs and heart exposed. It is imperative we protect our heart at all costs, especially physically. We all know our heart is not just an impressive four-chambered muscle the size of our fist. It has a mysterious component of emotions that is intangible as well, and it is the powerhouse of physical life. It is the seat of one's morality, which drives our good and bad passions in life. "A good man brings good things out of the good stored up in his heart, and an evil man brings evil things out of the evil stored up in his heart. For the mouth speaks what the heart is full of" (Luke 6:45). The human heart is so complex with its tangible and intangible components. It should be reserved for the dwelling place of the Lord—the Holy Spirit.

If we desire good things to be stored up in our hearts, we must have some divine help because we cannot be good and righteous all of the time on our own. Righteousness goes beyond just being good and moral, though. It has to do with an actual spiritual heart change that only God can provide. I like to define godly righteousness as just, equal, straight, and right before God. If we are at peace with God, clean from sin with a fully devoted and repentant heart, then our heart should seek beyond mere morality.

Morality is the beliefs about what is right behavior and what is wrong behavior.[6] Society has followed morality based on the current definition of good. When there are no laws or cultural barometers, we fail miserably. We need guidelines because our sin nature is so evil when left to its own demise. Think back to the days of Noah. His society fell so far from God's governance that God had to wash the sin away—literally. Genesis 6:11 tells the story as God declared to Noah, "I have determined to make an end of all flesh, for the earth is filled with violence through them" (Genesis 6:13, ESV).

A few decades ago, pornography was the farthest thing away from public television, but today it has slowly snuck its way onto primetime commercials of family shows. Our moral standards continue to decline every decade or less. "More than four out of five adults—83%—contend that they are concerned about the moral condition of the nation."[7]

Think back to 10 years ago. What shows were on television and to what extent did they have profanity, pornography, and marital affairs as their storyline? The changing morality of society will continue to decline because the heart of man is prone to evil (Genesis 8:21). Morality follows the standards of the current times and dictates what is currently permissible to

"The current morals of society are much different than the righteousness of God."

us—but God's standards do not change. God is the same yesterday, today, and forever (Hebrews 13:8). There is no guessing if God approves of something or not. All we have to do is read His Word and we will know where He stands.

Godly righteousness reflects the emotional and spiritual aspect of pleasing God through faith in Jesus. God set the standard of righteousness, which is timeless and unchanged. Righteousness is about being right before Him and having holy behavior, even when others are not looking.

There is an inward knowing in all of us between good and evil. We *know* when we do something wrong (James 4:17). This inner thought process declines when we continue to store up bad things in our hearts. We soon become numb to the gentle Holy Spirit nudges that tell us we are heading down the wrong path. If you are a believer in Christ, the Holy Spirit was given to you, within your heart, when you accepted Him. Jesus said the Holy Spirit will provide us with help and guidance (John 14:16, 26). Important evidence of the Holy Spirit in us is that we love others (Romans 5:5). We will fall short of loving everyone as Jesus does, but our goal is to increase and see growth in our love towards others.

I was never allowed to watch R-rated movies growing up, but many of my friends were, even though they were underage. Like most kids, we snuck things when parents were not looking. As adults, we can sneak things in when we think God is not looking too.

I distinctly remember the slumber party where I watched horror movies for the first time. I was terrified and disturbed at a whole new level. The enemy had a quick entrance into my heart with all the evil I was allowing in. The images stuck deep within me, ready to recall whenever the enemy wanted to use them in the future. I knew I was wrong for watching them, but at the next party, I repeated the sequence. I dismissed the check in my spirit because my heart had an inward pull to look at them again, even though I still knew it was not right. I did not tell my parents about it until after the images were downloaded in my mind. I had no idea how to arm myself or fight this cycle on my own.

If we want to clean up our insides and be righteous before God, we need to pray and ask the Holy Spirit to guide us, convict us, and remove us from the situation. We need to flee. Matthew 26:41 says that the heart of man is prone to being tempted. This proves that we have to be proactive about righteousness and that it is not going to come naturally or instinctively.

ARMOR ALERT: Getting It Right with God

Some habits can be hindrances because we cannot seem to remove them completely. Read the questions and spend a few minutes in prayer before answering.

1. **Is there anything you need to let go of from your past or present to march forward with Christ?**

2. **Ask Christ to forgive and cleanse you and help you move forward and not look back.** (See the end of this week for a sample prayer.)

Week 5, Day 2
Detox of the Heart

"But when you do a charitable deed, do not let your left hand know what your right hand is doing, that your charitable deed may be in secret; and your Father who sees in secret will Himself reward you openly."
—Matthew 6:3-4

When my husband and I were finishing our basement, the number one thing people told us to do was to leave even more space for storage—apparently, the two large closet areas did not seem to be enough. We cherished the wise counsel of friends, but both of us knew we were not hoarders. We chose not to take the advice and have lived these past 12 years happily with both large closets somewhat empty. We do not keep things that we do not need. When we receive mail, we immediately filter and trash what is not necessary because we find it incredibly liberating to let go, clean up, and throw things away. Just as we can clean out our junk drawers and detoxify our body, it is even more liberating when we accomplish this within our heart.

To detoxify our heart, we should recognize the toxins that need to be excavated. The Lord's Prayer in Matthew 6:12 says, "...forgive us our debts, as we also have forgiven our debtors." It reads past tense, meaning forgive us because we already have forgiven our neighbor. We cannot have deep cleansing when we are grappling with unforgiveness and bitterness. Matthew 5:22-24 tells us if we have an issue with someone, we must first be reconciled with them before coming to the Lord.

Detoxing our heart is not a one-time forgiveness session because chances are we are going to mess up again (maybe not in the same way, but we do not just completely stop sinning forever in this world). This is why Christ calls us to renew our minds daily and ask Him to cleanse us. We need Him every day, not just one day. When we come to the Lord with our sins, He forgives and cleanses us. It allows communication to heighten. When we obey the Lord, we listen and hear Him much clearer.

We are told to give to the poor and take in orphans. We are also directed to meet the needs of others in practical ways—like filling up a friend's gas tank, bringing a meal to a sick family, and mowing an elderly neighbor's lawn. When we bless others, something amazing happens inside. Our emotions ignite with an intangible satisfaction. Our hearts beat a little faster and we smile a little bigger. Righteousness is not just about making us feel good inside—that is just a blessing byproduct. Righteousness is a spiritual confirmation from God.

Who are we truly doing these blessings for—the "I," others, or God? "But when you do a charitable deed, do not let your left hand know what your right hand is doing, that your charitable deed may be in secret; and your Father who sees in secret will Himself reward you openly" (Matthew 6:3-4). We must ask ourselves what the condition of our heart is and what the motivation is for our good works; however, good works are not the only practice that makes us righteous.

God knows I have had ill feelings towards others. I have stood in gossip circles, and I've been known to cheat at cards back in the day. These too are all products of personal unrighteousness. These things do not seem as morally terrible as an evil act like stealing a car. They sure seem like smaller issues, and generally, have lesser consequences. However, they still count as unrighteousness toward God. This is the difference between righteousness and worldly standards. These minor daily sins do not appear to amount to much and are easily justifiable because we all do them, and more than we would like to admit. It's the norm to get away with the small stuff, so only the big offenses seem to be classified as unholy, unrighteous, or evil. However, God will show us the need to be cleansed from even these smaller offenses on His timeline. This is the gift of the Holy Spirit living on the inside, in the heart, of all those who believe (1 Corinthians 6:19, Romans 8:9). He desires to have our whole heart and not just part of it. He will help us chisel things away as needed.

In the nutrition world, one way to eliminate toxins from our physical body is to go through a cleanse or a detox. The definition of detoxify is to remove a poisonous or harmful substance from (something).[8] Not only can we detoxify our body, we can also detoxify our heart. This is why we have the Holy Spirit, to guide us and to show us where the cleanse needs to happen. To detox from the toxic stain, the sin, and the harm done, we only need to ask God.

"Fear the Lord and depart from evil. It will bring health to our flesh and strength to our bones" (Proverbs 3:8). I hear it often enough—"I'm not an evil person. I do some bad things from time to time, but nothing like murder or grand theft." Sin is sin, no matter how small—there are just different consequences of that sin. If we turn away from evil and cleave to Jesus, evil flees from our heart and our behavior changes—our heart changes. As we desire to heed Jesus' commands, the nudge of conviction from the Holy Spirit will be heard and will be much easier to obey. He helps us clean house in our hearts and even reveals things to us we never thought were issues. Conviction is a huge blessing. Without it there would never be a radical change.

ARMOR ALERT: Detoxification

1. **What smaller offenses do you need to detoxify from within your heart that might not seem as monumental as prison crimes?** (White lies, over-exaggerating, cheating, gossiping, non-committing, unforgiveness, being late, laziness, procrastinating, defaming, evil speaking, worrying, doubting, stinking thinking, negativity, jealousy, repetitive cravings, yes, it is hard to physically write these shortcomings in pen.)

2. What strategic action step can you take to arm yourself with righteousness?

3. God reveals His righteousness by:

- Instructing men in His Word (Psalm 25:8), or by priests, pastors, or prophets (Leviticus 10:11; Deuteronomy 4:1, 5, 14; 24:8).
- Fulfilling His promises (Nehemiah 9:1-8).
- Judging enemies (Exodus 9:27; Psalm 96:13) and even Israel (Ezekiel 9:15; 2 Chronicles 12:1-6).
- The way He rules (Psalm 45:6, 89:14, 97:2).
- His protection of the poor and afflicted (Psalm 140:12, 116:6).
- How He shows mercy and compassion (Psalm 116:5-6; Isaiah 30:18).
- His anger toward the wicked (Psalm 11:5, 7:11).

Trainer Talk

This 2-Week Emotional Challenge could be hard to get going, or even see measurable progress right away. Try not to treat it as a checklist, but rather a necessary goal you *will* reach. I have faith you can surpass your goals.

Week 5, Day 3
Organizing Your Desires

"Delight yourself also in the LORD, and He shall give you the desires of your heart. Commit your way to the LORD, trust also in Him, and He shall bring it to pass."
—Psalm 37:4-5

As a mom, there are countless areas in which I need to be strong and trust God—primarily regarding my family. However, it does not stop at just trusting. I still need to ask God for His plans in my situation, where and to whom I need to minister and give the most energy, how to organize my time with excellence, how to use my finances best, and then I need to obey the answer He gives. Wow, if it were that simple we would all be super moms. The enemy is at war trying to bait us with distractions, to steal our time from eternal progression. He is attacking our schedules and planting seeds of busyness to take our focus off our Godly assignments. Be on guard and be aware. He is prowling around seeking someone to destroy.

It is very easy to be over-committed in *good* things, and to be the "yes" girl, when we place our focus on lesser priorities. Often enough we enter areas we shouldn't go to in the first place, because we are so worn down. We can quickly find ourselves trying to hold the pieces together with glue that is not adhesive. Things just fall apart. We find we as equipped as we could be using caffeine, chocolate, or Grandma's pep talks for our daily energy source. God made women super strong in many ways, but think how much stronger we would be if we used God's strength as our source of energy.

"What if we focused on God's plans with excellence, instead of parading around with the "I" leading the way to self-ruin?"

As the world demands its fast-paced agenda, we reap the consequences of fast food, overdrawn checkbooks, lack of sleep and exercise, and barely enough left in the tank for quality family time. There just does not seem to be enough time for everything we want to do. Our coveted relationships are attacked right in front of us, and we appear helpless to stop it. The most important habits, agendas, and personal tasks are seen by the way we prioritize them. We will make time for what is important to us. I want God's plans with excellence, instead of parading around with the "I" leading the way to my self-ruin.

Have you ever wondered why we are so busy when we have so many modern devices, which are supposed to help us save time but actually do not? Washing machines, ovens and cars are daily convenient devices. With using just these three, we cut down many hours of time, yet seem to have less of it by the end of the day. Modern blessings allow us more time to do other things, but our other activities on which we choose to use the rest of our time is what is the focus. Are we taking any of this given time to relax, refresh, and rejuvenate, or are we cramming more things on our plates that are less important? We think we can do more and be successful at everything because we have this tiny spot on our plate that is still exposed.

Ladies, you are allowed to have an exposed spot on your plate. You need it, deserve it, and are called to it. The Bible says to be still and know He is God, a simple way to refresh your soul (Isaiah 28:12; Matthew 11:28-29).

Resting recharges and refocuses us. When focused, nothing is holding us back from accomplishing our God-given desires. God made us strong and amazingly capable of fulfilling any path set before us. Think for a moment on where your mind is focused most—things of this world or things of eternity? Relationships are forever. People are forever. Our designer jeans, make-up, and house will fade, along with our current physical bodies. Quality time spent with someone outlasts time spent on the "I" or in front of a screen. Is there anything eating your time without leaving spiritual fruit behind?

There may not be anything we need to take off our plate to find time to rest. We may just need to assess and prioritize what is currently on it. God can make all areas of our lives stronger and flow with balanced intention if we ask Him to lead us by His priorities. Some days we will not have time to do everything, but we can at least make sure we are doing things for and with God.

If you have ever felt a desire to apply for something, take up a hobby, join a new group, do something out of the ordinary, or go to a new place, this is not mere circumstance or coincidence. God gives us the desires of our heart (Psalm 37). The Holy Spirit places desires in our hearts for specific purposes to glorify God (Proverbs 4:11-13). He is at work; it is just up to us to listen and obey.

ARMOR ALERT: God's Strength or Your Own?

Take a moment to think about your obligations, relationships, free time, current purposes, and anything else to which you give your heart and time. Then answer the questions below.

1. **Is there something you are missing out because you are distracted with too many *good* things?**

2. **What action step can you take to help the situation?**

Week 5, Day 4
Commanded or Compelled?

"I have taught you in the way of wisdom; I have led you in right paths. When you walk, your steps will not be hindered, and when you run, you will not stumble. Take firm hold of instruction, do not let go; keep her, for she is your life."
—Proverbs 4:11-13

"Octopus? Is this really what we are having for dinner?" I questioned my health-conscious dad, who used to bring home some of the weirdest meal choices. He was what my siblings and I called a vitamin-aholic, a heavyweight lifter, and an expert on making banana chips in the oven. The average elementary kid and I thought the same—yuck. But, it was not just a suggestion from my dad to eat octopus, banana chips, and anything else placed in front of us. We were told—which means we had to do it. We do things out of respect, or out of obligation. My husband and I do not ask our kids to come to church with us—we tell them. There is no question come Sunday morning if we are going to sleep in or not. It might feel like an obligation to some of my kids, especially when they are exhausted from the week, but my hope is one day they will all feel compelled.

Many can place their right hand over their heart and pledge to a flag, but that does not mean they are a fully devoted follower of that promise. Merely going through the motions and giving lip service is a common practice even in some churches. If I command my kids to do something and never let them know why, their hearts may reject it due to a purposeless and stale obligation. Once we are older, our parental instruction would only be revered as a commanded childhood memory. The job of a parent is to train kids and help them along the straight and narrow path. If we do this by keeping their interests at the forefront of our teaching moments, it presents a more compelling reason to obey.

I attend church because I love God, and love brings commitment, reason, and purpose to my life. Think what life would be like without the love of God—void, barren, hopeless, and hated. These empty feelings are what the enemy provides because he is the exact opposite of God, and God is love. Think about the last time you experienced something that took your breath away; the feeling of a spontaneous kiss, the passionate warmth love imparts, the inside tingle of a whispered "I love you," when he got down on one knee, or your few moments leading up to the altar. Multiply the way you have experienced earthly love by one hundred, and it would be a mere taste of the presence of the Most High God's love for you. "But God shows his love for us in that while we were still sinners, Christ died for us" (Romans 5:8). If we think we can feel love through our relationships now, what do you suppose the root of love would ultimately be like when experiencing Him in heaven? There is no end to God's love (1 Corinthians 13).

The spiritual forces behind the scenes will try to bait you with immense doubt so that you question the love He has for you. If you have never given your fully devoted allegiance to the King of all Kings, now is the time to ask why. Would God really have His Son tortured and killed if there were another way? He is not what society labeled as just another religious leader. He was and is more powerful and holds the highest level of authority over all religions, masters, kings, lords and leaders because He conquered the very spiritual conquest none of them ever could—death.

Death is final for all human leaders. They have no authority to bypass it. No other rock star, self-proclaimed billionaire, or political leader can come close to Jesus' unfailing love for humanity. None of them died in the place of their followers, bore the weight of sin, and returned to the earth to tell of it in person. This is the most amazing love story ever given, and it is available to anyone who seeks it.

God is interested in our hearts and should be the reason we go to church, pray, serve, and love others. When love is interwoven with commitment, we are compelled to run after it, without seeing it as a command. If your purpose in life or your relationship with God feels obligatory or dry and you desire one that is more compelling, you have the most incredible opportunity to renew and refresh your walk with Him. It is not just reorganizing your schedule that is exciting. You can have your relationship with the King of Kings ignited to a new level with driven force and excitement. It is one of the most liberating feelings to know God's will and be compelled to run after Him.

God is available right now for you. He tells us to ask Him anything. He loves you more deeply than any relationship you have on earth—now that is love! Ask Him to fill you with His greater purposes, many adventures, exciting moments, and to help you walk with Him in a compelling and loving relationship.

ARMOR ALERT: Divine Goals

1. **Are you compelled, sold out, or excited to follow God? Why or why not?**

2. **What current assignment or adventure is He leading you on?**

Before You Meet

Put on the Breastplate of Righteousness

Moment for Meditation (Use your own words or this as a sample.)

Father,

I put on the belt of truth and ask to have truth braced around my core at all times. Give me wisdom about Your Word and open my eyes to see what You are telling me.

I put on the breastplate of righteousness. Protect me from the enemy and make me aware of moral declines within my heart. Forgive me of my sins, big and small. Cleanse my heart from every last bit of unrighteousness. Help me detoxify from (name them).

Help me be strong and stand for what is right—even if that means standing alone. Give me holy behavior. Help me be righteous even when no one is looking. I pray Your full armor over me and my family; gird my waist with truth, my heart with righteousness, my mind with your salvation, my feet with your Gospel and peace, and shield me with great faith.

Help me to read and understand your Word with help from the Holy Spirit. Fulfill Your Godly righteousness in my life.

Thank You for cleansing me and making me right in Your eyes. Amen.

IT'S TIME TO MEET!

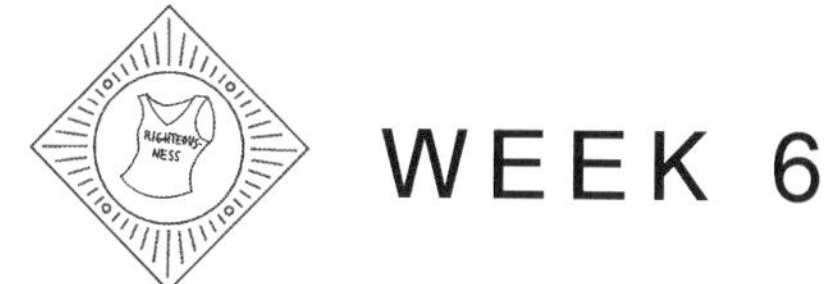

WEEK 6

ARM YOURSELF WITH EMOTIONAL HEALTH

Week 6, Day 1
Emotional Wars

"And the LORD, He is the One who goes before you. He will be with you, He will not leave you nor forsake you; do not fear nor be dismayed."
—Deuteronomy 31:8

When one of my kids wakes up on the wrong side of the bed, it is not uncommon for the whole family to reap the frustrations and tension floating in the air from that one grumpy child. Of course, the siblings do not help when they retaliate in irritation. This silly war can start within two minutes into the morning routine. When we do not intervene as parents, the day begins with a bust and the battle rages on with contempt in their hearts. These little fires in our hearts can make us engage in the wrong war with each other quickly. We feel entitled to participate because others treat us poorly. This disrupts our emotional health as we allow these little squabbles to steal our joy.

Every woman has emotions; we just do not express them the same. We can loudly share them, keep them moderately surfaced as needed, or stuff them down deep. Emotion can be defined as a conscious mental reaction (such as anger or fear) subjectively experienced as strong feeling usually directed toward a specific object and typically accompanied by physiological and behavioral changes in the body.[9] Love compels us to smile more during our day. When cherished, we have a sense of improved self-worth and hold our heads up higher, as we do with promotions, positive recognitions, or the feelings of achieving our health goals.

When emotions are attacked, our behavior can be anything but holy as we decide what response plan to use. This is the point where we can easily engage in the wrong battle when we are not prepared. It is easy to lower our guard and look to the "I" instead of God. Frankly, this is because God does not work the way we do. He has us do things like wait, or look the other way, or even be silent and keep pressing forward. If we decline to obey God and allow sin to enter in, it is like allowing the enemy to draw his bow, point the flaming arrow at our hearts, and release. The enemy will use his tactics to stir the pot by baiting us with simple nuances from others because these can turn into full-blown relationship wars. A simple smirk from an acquaintance can do more damage than an overflowed toilet. When we protect our hearts with Godly righteousness, these silly things will not matter. Perspectives shift and the things of this world fade—especially drama from other women. Keeping sin from our hearts and seeking righteousness won't allow us to enter the wrong battles unarmed.

The wars God commanded in the Old Testament are a great example for us today. God had specific purposes pertaining to the Promised Land with the Israelites—it held a unique and vital place in salvation history. The possession of the land was dependent on Israel's faithfulness (1 Samuel 17; 2 Chronicles 20). Of the battles recorded in the Old Testament, 42 were won, and 19 were lost. What should not come as a surprise is that when Israel was faithful to God they won, and when they went out on their own and followed the "I," they were defeated. We might not be in physical wars, but the principle of the story is clear.

We have all had friendship wars at one time or another. They are taxing, emotional, very disruptive to our everyday lives, and they steal our joy. I pondered why they mean so much and why they affect us so deeply. The greatest commandments are to love God with all our heart and love our neighbor as our self. If these are the two greatest commandments, our relationships would then be a logical place for the enemy to attack. Satan's goal is to kill, steal, and destroy. He will attack our relationships with force. He wants to rip apart our friendships forever, especially those closest to us. This is the war we should focus on and engage in, not the little squabbles from others. We do this through a clean heart with God in prayer.

A while back a friend wounded me deeply, but I realized that after her apology, I was still unforgiving in my heart. I prayed for peace and a means to be released from my emotional battle, but none was given at the time. I was asking God amiss. I pleaded with Him to take away my hurt instead of my bitterness. I felt entitled to hang on to the bitterness because the hurt ran deep. This battle was raging within me. I allowed my spirit to engage in a war with me, myself, and the "I." When I decided to come clean with God, seek repentance from my bitterness, and forgive her, is when I finally saw victory in my battle.

Just as Israel's victories came from God, ours will too. Communicating with God, regardless if in physical, emotional, or mental struggles, must be on the forefront of our hearts. The Promised Land conquests are a great example for us to follow instead of the "I." We need to allow Him to go before and after the "I," asking Him to show us what, when, and how to engage. When we do not, the "I" creates holes in our spiritual armor, exposing our hearts. Our relationships can bring joy or doom and must be actively pursued and protected. They cannot be left on autopilot without investing in them.

ARMOR ALERT: Holy Emotions

1. **Is there an emotional battle within your soul?** (Inadequacy, fear, doubt, worry, bitterness, relationship, frustration, etc.)

2. What is one action step you are willing to take today to combat it?

Week 6, Day 2
Emotional Jealousy

"A sound heart is life to the body, but envy is rottenness to the bones."
—Proverbs 14:30

Some may feel their insides warm up just by reading the title of the day—possibly because there is a personal issue with these gripping words. It does not matter if you are an emotional person or not; jealousy disrupts our health in two major ways—emotionally and mentally. But it sure does not stop with the majors. Jealousy disrupts us socially and, given tim; it will disrupt us physically. Jealousy can strip us of everything and hold us in bondage to vulnerability. I know this all too well because this title sure had a grip on me.

I distinctly remember a particular chapel service in college because it was all devoted to overcoming jealousy. To the average person, I was anything but jealous. In fact, it looked on the outside that I had everything going for me. *Why would I be jealous of anything?* I did not covet things and my needs were met. This is where it all started. The "I" did not need anything and the "I" had everything. I looked too much from within, and not enough at Christ. I knew deep down inside the "I" filled me was running the show in my life more than God.

The chapel speaker said the average person is gripped to the core by this emotional trickery. This was when I became uneasy inside. I thought about fleeing the chapel service of 5,000 students, but then it would clearly show guilt. I stuck to my chair. When I realized I had an overwhelming desire for the speaker to stop talking, it hit me. I had a deep issue with jealousy. It was tearing me apart inside as I sat in my seat.

I quickly decided I did not like the speaker because he kindly asked all those who were struggling with jealousy to first admit to ourselves there was an issue by standing, and second, to admit it before God by coming forward. My heart started beating faster within my chest. To my amazement, it seemed like the entire sanctuary got up and went to the altar, except me, and the few others possibly dealing with the same internal drama. The freeing feeling I wished I could have was just a few steps of acceptance away, yet I sat super-glued in my chair. My heart pounded louder in my chest. I was clearly experiencing physical symptoms from an emotional issue, proving to me personally that this was a spiritual battle with spiritual roots. My heart was drumming louder, but the "I" was even louder and made me unmovable. My brain could not connect the dots to make my physical body stand. The emotional agony I felt when I left the building was beyond dreadful.

I remember that day so clearly because it followed me like bad baggage for years. I felt as if my bones were rotting inside, consuming my thoughts and my physical body. I was not armed properly and ready to battle the fiery pride monster. I wanted to be free, but not badly enough that I would expose my inadequacies. The "I" kept winning as jealousy spread like raging cancer. It would seem to go in remission but would come back when I least expected.

Jealousy is a gripping force, waging war and spreading its cause. Even though I prayed individually many times, even on my knees, it did not escape me. I wanted freedom without the cost of losing my pride. As the months turned into years, I stuffed it deep and accepted it as something that would just be a part of my life.

Jealousy means to have an unhappy or angry feeling of wanting to have what someone else has. Jealousy is the cousin to covetousness.[10] The Ten Commandments clearly state—do not covet (Exodus 20:17). God knows if we desire something long enough, we will break other commandments. King David sent his friend to the front lines in battle to ensure his death, which meant he could marry his dead friend's beautiful wife. I cannot imagine any of us sending someone to death like this, but I will be the first to admit I have wished that a certain individual, who hurt me deeply, would not be around me anymore.

"Jealousy is a gripping force, waging war and spreading its cause."

I have been so envious of another person's so-called "perfect" body that I have disliked that person. I have talked to many women who have unfortunately felt the same. Some are jealous of a car, a house, or an outfit. What about another person's spouse, a friend's relationship with God, or the spiritual gifts of another? I did not like the chapel presenter when he spoke on jealousy, and I did not even know the guy. I was engaged in a distasteful battle that was all about me. It had nothing to do with who God chose as the mouthpiece to reveal my sin. Being jealous of someone is very hard to overcome, trust me. But God is stronger than our issues and can free us from anything.

Some sins are harder to extinguish than others. There are times we need help from friends who will pray with us, or a humble and freeing trip to the altar in front of others. Other times what we need is the perfect timing of God's intervention in the quietness of our home.

Was I being punished for not getting up out of my pew so many years ago? God is just, and there are consequences to our disobedience. Consequence and justice both produce better returns in the end. God was merciful and forgiving, but I still had to be active and admit my sins.

Years later, a message on jealousy was delivered in a church service. My heart began pounding louder than the pastor was speaking. I thought others could hear it. I sat on the edge of my seat waiting for the pastor to say the words I longed to hear. I knew he was going to ask us to come to the altar—my second chance to be free from jealousy. The freedom that I had been longing for was waiting for me. I was the first to jump out of my seat. I did not care what others thought. I was not going to wait any longer and let this eat away at me. I wanted the grip to be loosed right then—and it was, thanks to Jesus!

Jealousy can still get the best of me when I am not focused on God, but it no longer has a grip on me. When we sit still long enough to communicate and listen to the Holy Spirit's conviction (John 16:8) and repent with all honesty and humility, freedom is present.

ARMOR ALERT: Jealous Anyone?

Pray that God puts graciousness on your lips and sweetness in your heart. Ask God to fill you with unconditional love for everyone. Remember, this is one of His commandments, to love others. Are you jealous of others, even a tiny bit? Maybe certain situations or people are popping up in your mind?

1. **Fill in names of people, situations, or things you are jealous of. Then, make this list part of your prayer life. Be honest with yourself and before God.** (It is hard to hate or be jealous when you are praying for someone.)
    a.
    b.
    c.
    d.

2. **Take a few moments to pray these spiritual applications to combat jealousy:**
    a. Ask God to intervene (Romans 8:26; 1 John 5:14; Jude 1:20).
    b. Confess any sin, known and unknown (James 5:16; 1 John 1:9).
    c. Recognize of whom you are jealous and pray blessings for them (Matthew 5:43-48; Luke 6:27).
    d. Speak to that person if you have a conflict (Matthew 18:15-17, 5:9; Ephesians 4:29).
    e. Understand you are not alone in this fight with jealousy (Isaiah 41:10; Deuteronomy 31:6).
    f. Always remember to pray (1 Thessalonians 5:17; James 5:16).

Trainer Talk

Nothing is impossible with God. God wants you to succeed in all that you do. He asks that you do all things as if doing them for Him. Does your 2-Week Challenge have Christ at the center of it? If you feel emotional during your days ahead, remember you can put on the breastplate of righteousness. You can ask God to open your heart to specific truths that you need at that very moment. He can bring peace to a situation when there doesn't seem to be any. Make it a priority to go to Him first.

Week 6, Day 3
Emotional Addictions

"Draw near to God, and He will draw near to you."
—James 4:8a

When we feel a craving coming on and allow it to take up more than a few seconds in our thoughts, something strange happens. We visualize ourselves doing it. It is like a trailer to a great movie. We see scene snippets of ourselves being hungry, heading to the drive-thru, looking at the menu, and deciding what to eat. What is worse is after we visualize this internal trailer, somehow our physical car steers itself right into the closest drive-thru. We find ourselves helpless to drive away from the ordering line. We place our order and the movie is now unfolding. If these moments are not immediately conquered, they will do more damage than puckering and dimpling our buttocks. They will pull us into a drive-thru of the heart. Cravings do not just attack us through our food.

"If we did not crave anything, we would feel no need for Him because we would be satisfied with the 'I.'"

The repeating cycle of inadequate cravings soon becomes an emotional tug-of-war. We conquer them sometimes, but not nearly as much as we should. When we notice our bodies growing out of our clothes, we know very well there is an expanding problem behind it. Cellulite slowly surfaces to show the body needs physical attention. Cellulite is a by-product of food cravings, and by the way, we all have it—even me. We also know how it got there. These physical desires are not coming from our stomach. Many are emotional triggers that attach themselves to us with deep-seeded claws, which are not easy to shake off. If we allow the movie trailer to be played in the first place, we will generally act on it. Once we devote more time and money to it, we are emotionally attached and quickly fall prey to addiction.

Cravings are not always wrong. When I am thirsty, I crave water. This leads to health, not obesity. When hurt by a friend, I crave reconciliation, which leads to restoration. When I am cold, I crave heat, which makes me physically comfortable. God blessed us with desires and cravings and tells us He will give us the desires of our hearts. If we truly need physical intimacy and are married, our husband is that provider. Above any craving or addiction, we need spiritual intimacy with God.

In our culture, the word intimacy has become synonymous with sex. We may think we need physical intimacy most, but we need spiritual oneness with God. We must come to Him in truth. God is Spirit (John 4:24). The roots of our cravings are not the manifestation we physically act out; they are the hidden reasons behind those actions, like insecurity, depression, or lack of intimacy with God.

God allowed us to crave things so we could ultimately love and desire Him. If we did not crave anything, we would feel no need for Him because we would be satisfied with the "I." There are consequences for craving and being addicted to the wrong things. If there were no implications for eating sugar, why wouldn't everyone be eating it constantly?

ARMOR ALERT: Cravings

1. **List your emotional cravings** (Specific foods or drinks, appearances, sex, closeness, acceptance, love, true friends, being cherished and honored, shopping, medication, drugs, etc.)

2. **Take time to identify what is hindering you from conquering any of the above.** (Time, schedule, resources, encouragement, money, passion, accountability, loneliness, apathy, obedience, relationships, intimacy, discipline, etc.)

3. **What is one action step you can take to reverse harmful cravings?**

Week 6, Day 4
Emotional Remembrances

"Remember now your Creator in the days of your youth, before the difficult days come, and the years draw near when you say, 'I have no pleasure in them'."
—Ecclesiastes 12:1

Our church teenagers just returned from a memorial month of missions work and came to my house to tell me all about it. It was especially exciting to hear from those who experienced God for the first time and found their own faith, instead of living off the coattails of their parents' faith. I was excited to see their zeal for the Lord. It was contagious. After I had heard oodles of stories and experiences, I asked them if they wrote anything down. Although an adult on the mission trip told them to write everything down as well, none of them had.

It is amazing how we forget the good moments even from yesterday. I have a farmer friend that raises sheep. I never realized how dumb sheep were until I heard the stories. I knew sheep were not the brightest animal in the barn, but these little animals do not even know how to retreat from danger. My friend's lamb got its little head stuck in barbed wire. It did not have the capacity to remember that it was in danger. I am an outsider to the whole farm thing, but it was to me that if the lamb would just back up a few inches, it would be free. This proves how much I don't know sheep. It just kept charging forward as if it would free itself by going through the small circle. It ended up dying. Sheep are dependent on a leader, their very own shepherd who they distinctly hear above all others. I now understand why God gave us a Shepherd and why He calls us His sheep—as humbling as that is.

I have found through the years when I wonder off and am not listening to my Shepherd daily, my mind speaks to my heart in ways I do not care for. It is like it only seems to drudge up hurtful memories. Why does it not recall the memories that gave me joy? Thoughts that damaged my heart most apear to linger longest. They momentarily overshadow anything that is positive. We can turn to the negative and forget about the positive all too quickly. This is why it is a great action step to write things down that are positive. It is when I listen and follow my Shepherd that He captures me and reminds me of the good. This is when bad memories begin to fade.

I was told by a friend to keep a prayer journal, one in which I could write down my prayers, date them, and record how they were answered. I accepted this task. I was surprised after a few months when I looked back. Every prayer was answered. Now, I did not say the prayers were answered how I wanted, but they were with either yes or no, or in a totally different way than I expected. It was fascinating to look back at. I now know the reason why some of them were answered with a no, instead of them being answered my way. God knows the bigger picture, and I learned to trust Him with the decisions, even though I do not always agree or like it at the moment.

I was also challenged to write down my God-moments, just like I told the teenagers to do. I recorded so many thoughts, the way God answered my prayers, people I planted Gospel seeds with, and even the way I saw God intervene in situations. I did not write them all down (I wish I would have now), but if I had not written any down, I would not be able to recall them all. Remember, we are compared to sheep. As I look back and read over my highlighted times, those damaging and stressed moments pale in comparison to all the good and joyful ones. I not only have to renew my mind with Christ daily, but I also enjoy renewing my emotions with the good in my life.

If I am watching or listening to the evening news, almost all of it is negative. Every once in a while there is a story that leaves me feeling a little refreshed and uplifted, but generally speaking, this is not the case. What is drawing us in to hear the bad instead of the good? If there were a news station dedicated only to good reports, it wouldn't earn nearly the ratings as the normal stations do. People want to hear bad stories so they have something to talk about, just like gossip. K-LOVE radio station has God-based stories all the time on the air. It is uplifting and encourages others. It takes the edge off people while they are driving to work and fills them with hope for at least a moment. Look for the positives as much as possible.

ARMOR ALERT: Remembering the Good Times

1. **Do you tend to listen more to emotional baggage from others or encouraging stories?**

2. **Write a few God-moments or stories so you can remember and share them with your AP.** (I encourage you to buy a journal and write down your emotional victorious moments, so you'll never forget them.)

Testimony

In the first year of our marriage, my husband and I lost two babies to miscarriage. Our hearts were broken. My emotions and body were ravaged. I endured three D&Cs and my body took 5 months to re-regulate itself. To make matters worse, my husband and I dealt with our pain differently. I was an emotional talker and he was quietly stuffing his pain. I felt alone and unsupported. I was 33 years old, barren and intensely jealous and angry when I would see expectant mothers or happy young families. I did not understand why this was happening to us, or what I had done wrong. I blamed God for my pain and so I began running as far away from Him as possible.

Heartbroken and fearing we may never have children of our own, we became a licensed foster/adopt family in 2007. This process was brutal. We were scrutinized meticulously, all for the sake of being deemed "qualified" to have children. I understand the need for this, but having done no wrong except my body not cooperating, it felt deeply personal.

After six months I became pregnant for a third time. It was at this point I returned to church in the hopes I could somehow influence the outcome in my favor, still believing to some degree that God was punishing me. My pregnancies were not easy and I arranged for medical intervention. In July 2008, our son Grant was born, then 15 months later, our daughter Hope followed.

It took a while for church to be more than just a means to an end, but I had always been involved heavily in my church and knew I would raise my children in a Christian home. In my heart, I always knew God loved me and had His best in store for me. With the love and support of friends and some counseling, I finally came to terms with the losses and realized that while nothing I experienced was "OK," I was OK. Ben and Ava are in the presence of God. Their father and I will see them again! Mommy loves you!

Dawn Olson
Bettendorf, IA

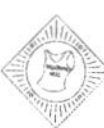

Before You Meet

These past two weeks we focused on our emotional health. These topics could be a little closer to some women's hearts, thus sharing could be a little harder than normal. There may be some emotional memories that surface that may be hard to articulate or share. A great opportunity to pray for your meeting with your AP. What nuggets have helped most with your nutrition?

It is that time again to do a quick review of your Pre-Evaluation Chart.

Left side of chart: sad, uncontrolled, weary, worn, jealous, judgmental, angry, depressed, unstable, closed-off, unrighteous in anger, selfish, entitled, toxic, unholy, afraid, shameful

Right side of chart: happy, confident, stable, joyful, controlled, even tempered, peaceful, easy going, forgiving, a goal-setter, courageous, positive, obedient, building character

Trainer Talk

When you underline words above, does it make it more concrete? Does it seem like it's more real and humbling? Talk to your AP and ask her how she progressed through her 2-Week Emotional Challenge. It's your job to check in and ask the hard questions (remember, she gave you permission). When the going gets tough, put on your breastplate of righteousness, with the Holy Spirit.

Remember to look your AP in her eyes and tell her how thankful you are that she is in your life. Fill and fuel her emotional tank with your appreciation.

IT'S TIME TO MEET!

SECTION FOUR

GOSPEL OF PEACE

This section pushes forward with the next two weeks focusing on how the Gospel and peace correlate to our social health. Our lives revolve around relationships. For most, it is the core of our daily interaction. Other people are the reason why we love this life so much. We communicate in many different avenues, and one thing we should always be communicating is the Gospel of Jesus—either verbally or non-verbally.

We are the hands and feet of Jesus in a lot of ways; talking, writing, giving, serving, loving, listening, etc. We will not always the mouthpiece. We do not have to witness the Gospel with our lips. We are told to witness, and that happens in many different ways. There is not one formula for everyone. Some people will plant a seed of the Gospel and others may water or harvest it.

Our job is to communicate the love and peace of Jesus and to try to do it like Him. Because relationships are interwoven, and quite intricate, they can be hard to manage at times. Frankly, relationships can get messy. I find it harder to share the Gospel to a family member than a stranger. We will never be perfect in our relationships all the time, so use this section to help make them even more amazing. I am super excited and hope you will take some of these nuggets on the following pages with you in your relationships and when you witness.

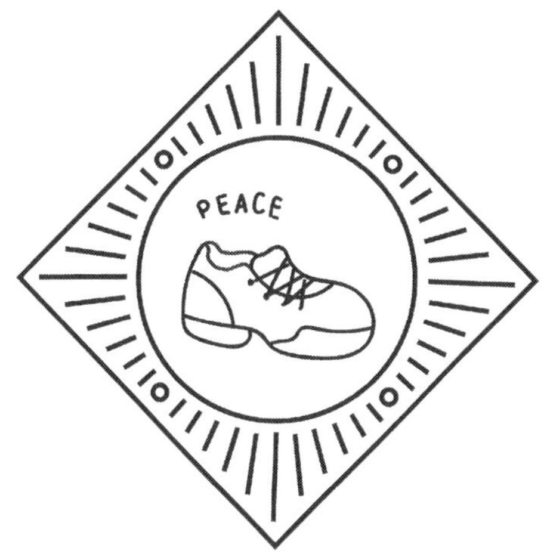

Week 7: Arm Yourself with Peace
Week 8: Arm Yourself with Social Health

Health Challenge #4
2-Week Relationship Challenge

When presented with challenges, we can look through different colored glasses. I might need to work more on my spiritual application for this challenge—loving others when they seem to be unlovable—while others may apply this challenge through serving more. Whatever the pair of glasses you will look through, your challenge is to try to strengthen your relationships. You might use it towards your spouse, children, co-worker, friend, or a combination.

1. Go a whole day without complaining to a particular person—then try for another day, etc.
2. Turn off all electronics when around others. Engage in conversation instead.
3. Create a new rule at your house not to have technology while eating, while driving in the car with others, after 9 PM, etc. Be intentional with conversation.
4. Do not place anything negative on social media for two whole weeks.
5. If you begin negative talk in your mind about someone, immediately pray for that person and ask God to fill you with love for them.
6. Engage in a few deeper than normal conversations.
7. Seek forgiveness the right way; be the first one to do it, admit to that person what you did, apologize for it, and then ask them to forgive you.
8. Seek out someone you have meant to get together with, set a time, and place to meet.
9. Encourage someone who needs it—practically, spiritually, emotionally, mentally, or financially.
10. Treat your children as a good co-worker. Do not yell, belittle, demean, exasperate, or be rough with them, but rather respect and honor them, listening to them.
11. Respect and honor your leadership by a random act of kindness.
12. Invite someone new to your church, to the gym, or to do something with you.
13. Do something out of normalcy with your social health—join a book club, gym, fitness class, sewing club, cooking club, take art or dancing lessons, talk to a checkout clerk, or invite someone over for dinner.
14. Encourage someone else in a big way, such as a surprise dinner, offering to babysit their kids, buy their tickets, invite them to something they cannot afford, etc.
15. Pray for specific relationships daily. Write down what you are praying for.

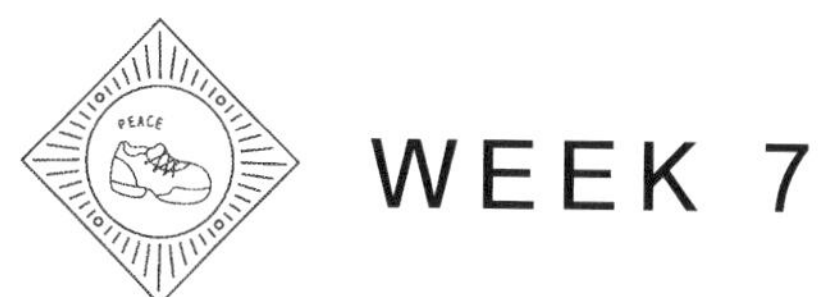

WEEK 7

ARM YOURSELF WITH PEACE

Week 7, Day 1

Gospel of Peace

"Stand therefore, having girded your waist with truth, having put on the breastplate of righteousness, and having shod your feet with the preparation of the gospel of peace."
—Ephesians 6:14-15

The Gospel of peace is one of my favorite pieces of armor because this is an action piece. We can know many aspects of the spiritual war and the Gospel, but if we do not put action behind coming against the enemy, it is of no effect. In order to shod our feet with the Gospel of peace, we must know and believe what the Gospel truly is.

We do not use the word "shod" in social conversations these days. When we physically shod our feet, we put on a type of footgear, such as shoes. Spiritually speaking, the Bible calls us to put on peace and take the Gospel with us wherever our feet lead us. This is done in numerous ways, and since the Lord works in mysterious ways, it is very exciting to see and experience how this is achieved.

This Good News (the Gospel) is not to be stored up in our hearts, without sharing it with others. Jesus tells us all to share our faith (Mark 16:15), but we are not all told to witness in the same way. You may feel like yelling it from mountain peaks, while others share Jesus through spending time with someone. Witnessing can involve evidence, testimony, and attestation through smiles, listening, giving gifts, or meeting practical needs. The possibilities of how to share the Gospel are endless. When we witness about Jesus, we are testifying about our relationship with Him, giving evidence of His existence, and proving our love for Him within our spirit. No one can refute our personal testimonies or our relationship statuses with someone else, whatever the relationship level. It belongs to us personally.

Sometimes there is a problem when we share our relationship with Jesus to others. It can be bothersome to people who do not yet believe. Not everyone we share our faith with will believe and accept in "simple" faith. The enemy does not want anyone to proclaim or accept Christ, so he places spiritual barriers and antagonists that try to stop the progression of it.

If you shared news of your grandma who has cancer with a close friend, you might have a hard time doing it because it is personal. However, there would not be resistance to accepting the news from the listener because they would not refute your feelings. The friend would validate the truth of your personal situation merely by your words alone. There would be no further action required from your friend because they believe your personal testimony. Since our relationship with Christ is not just emotional but has spiritual impact, unbelievers cannot just take or leave the Gospel information we give. By sharing our faith in Jesus Christ, it makes them have to take action by either accepting or rejecting the message. This is why some are offended or angry when we share. If they decide to believe, they have to change the way they live.

"A heart at peace is life to the body."—Proverbs 14:30

Accepting this relationship could cost them comfortable freedoms that seem better than God's rules and statutes. It would shake up possible social outlets, friendships, and daily living. This is a huge mental shift, emotional change, and spiritual decision that some will not accept immediately because the price tag seems too high. The cost is not worth the displacement of the "I," and so the spiritual unrest rages on within them, or they try to block it out as much as they can.

I have shared the Gospel with many who have immediately embraced it with both arms open wide—especially children. It was as if they could not wait to receive it. However, adults take a little longer to accept the truth of Jesus because they need to count the cost, sift through their mental warehouse of what is permissible, and seek out more proof—just as Thomas did in the Bible. He needed to physically see Jesus' pierced hands and feet. If you are unsure of what you truly believe, take the time and find out. If you know what you believe, my encouragement to you is this—have patience with the friend who needs more time to count the cost. Speak peacefully, and without contempt. Share this message with love. God calls us to share the Gospel with peace. Consistently pray for the listener that God would show them whatever proof they need.

I was deeply grieved as a child when my friend would not accept the Gospel of Jesus. She began to resent me, dislike me, and soon made fun of me. I thought it was how I said it or that I messed up sharing Jesus altogether. I later learned it had nothing to do with me, the messenger. She rejected the Gospel message—Jesus. Some will not accept regardless of how we say it. It could be it's not just the right time.

"Dear children, let us not love with words or speech but with actions and in truth" (1 John 3:18). Some missionaries have gone to unknown tribes where God has shown up to help communicate the Gospel in mysterious ways. Some of these mysterious ways had nothing to do with verbal communication, but rather through serving and ministering to their basic needs. Some husbands are won over to Christ by their wife's dedication to reading the Bible every day. Our non-verbal witness is at times more precious than our vocal megaphone. Peace comes when harmony surrounds relationships. If we love others, walking in peace comes naturally, and as does our message of the Cross.

Many of us have shared the Gospel by being hospitable and meeting physical needs with clothing, food, shelter, or through good deeds (Matthew 5:16). Some of us have prayed privately, given a listening ear, or brought over a meal with a note of encouragement. No matter our place, style, or method of witnessing, we can win people over to Christ through the Holy Spirit's leading if we bring it with peace.

ARMOR ALERT: Have You Acted?

1. Do you enjoy or struggle sharing your faith vocally?

2. Have you ever witnessed someone else sharing the Gospel in a hostile way?

3. I challenge you to seek God's plan for witnessing or ministering to someone else this week. Then share your experience with your AP.

Week 7, Day 2
Running Wildly

"Therefore go and make disciples of all nations, baptizing them in the name of the Father, and the Son and of the Holy Spirit."
—Matthew 28:19

I often think I will die when old and gray, and possibly a little later than the average life expectancy because I took good care of my physical body. Most of us feel we will live a long life. I think many feel they will live a long life, but feelings do not always come true. The fact is, we will breathe our last breath one day, and we do not believe it is coming anytime soon. I cannot help but think of the person I am supposed to share my faith with that does not have as long to live like me. 1 Thessalonians 5:12 tells us He will come for His children like a thief in the night. This should make us want to share, encourage, and bring to faith those with whom we are called to share the Gospel—with excitement and fear.

Sometimes I miss the opportunity to share my faith, big time. I can get too busy, with too much internal noise to hear that *still small voice* inside. This is not the "I" we are talking about, but the Holy Spirit. It is a quiet beckoning at what seems like the most inconvenient times, like running after a stranger. Usually, this is how the Holy Spirit communicates with me—quietly in my heart, like a prompting in my gut that I need to do something, and at times I do not expect. Whenever He hands us instructions for battle, we need to obey no matter if He says stay, wait, or go immediately. If we hesitate, we could miss something so wonderful.

I am an avid runner and train for many different types of races. Last summer, my general running schedule woke me up naturally around 5 AM on most mornings. I would wake up before my alarm because I yearned to run (it's called the runner's high). I loved being out as the birds were waking and the sun was breaking all signs of night. It was peaceful, and there were not too many gas fumes penetrating my lungs from cars yet. One particular morning was different. I remember lying in bed trying to guess how many more minutes until my alarm would sound, when all of a sudden, I had this overwhelming urge to find this lady on my running route and witness to her. I just knew it was that still small voice inside urging me in my spirit to act immediately.

I jumped out of bed, laced up my sneakers, and soon was running intently as I searched for her. Then it hit me—I had no conversation plan if I found her. Then, immediately, I knew. I was supposed to ask her if she had Jesus as her personal Savior. I do not mind witnessing, but this was a different one for me—running after a stranger? After a few miles, I thought I must have missed the internal message. I started second guessing myself. I was pretty sure this lady was the one, but maybe I missed the timing. As I began my run back home, as if out of thin air, there she was on the sidewalk heading right for me. I gained some ground, and my heart began to beat faster—that nervous beat when you know you have to do something you really do not want to do but know you have to do it. I got closer, but instead of stopping, I just kept running. I did not stop. I could not believe it. It was as if a muzzle was slapped over my mouth and my feet were on autopilot. Immediately, deep in my soul, I felt as if I let someone down who was counting on me. It was an overwhelming regret within my heart.

I prayed and asked God for confidence to try again. I turned around to go after her. I had to pick up the pace. I then knew if I did not sprint after her, I would lose her. Right before I caught up with her, she stopped and turned around. She asked if I was following her. I told her I was and explained how God wanted me to tell her He loves her. I asked if she went to church. She replied she did. We had a little more conversation and then I began my run home.

On my trot home, I realized I did not exactly do what God asked me to. I was relieved I partly obeyed and stopped the walker, but I only followed half of His plan. I did not ask her if she had a relationship with Jesus Christ as her personal Savior. I knew I was supposed to ask that specific question, and I missed it. This was a test from God. As I ran home, I repented and asked Him to increase my faith to be more obedient.

A few weeks later at a Bible study, we were to give accounts for ways God used us. I told the group my experience with the sidewalk lady. Not more than a week or so later, my pastor's wife said the sidewalk woman wrote about her experience with me in the paper—she just happened to be a columnist for our local paper. She wrote about a young lady (I am glad I am still considered young) who stopped her on the streets to talk about God, and that it challenged her so much she went home and read her Bible. She described life in this column as a sandwich. There are different things we can put in it—lettuce (kids), pickles (sports), meat (job)—that are all sandwiched together. But, most do not find room for God in their super-sized sandwich. She went on to say she was encouraged and she was going to make more room for God in her life.

God honored my confession of not doing exactly what He called me to do, yet provided a follow up that confirmed His blessing on my partial obedience. What a cool Father.

ARMOR ALERT: Running Out of Your Way

1. **Have you ever gone out of your way to witness for Christ? If so, please share with your AP.**

2. **Pray and ask God to give you (more) opportunities to witness and that you would have the courage to obey.**

Week 7, Day 3

Actions are Louder than Megaphones

"But I say to you who hear, love your enemies, do good to those who hate you, bless those who curse you, pray for those who abuse you. To one who strikes you on the cheek, offer the other also, and from one who takes away your cloak do not withhold your tunic either. Give to everyone who begs from you, and from one who takes away your goods do not demand them back."
—Luke 6:27-30, ESV

I love the story of "Les Miserable," the French historical novel by Victor Hugo. It is considered one of the greatest novels of the 19th-century. The main thread is the story of ex-convict Jean Valjean, who becomes a force for good in the world after his poor past. He is released from 19 years of imprisonment and is turned away by innkeepers because his passport marks him as a former convict. The benevolent Bishop Myriel gives him shelter. However, Valjean runs off with Myriel's silverware. When the police capture Valjean, the Bishop pretends he has given the silverware to Valjean and presses him to take two silver candlesticks as well as if Valjean had forgotten to take them. The police accept his story. Myriel tells Valjean that his life was spared for God, that he should use the silver candlesticks to make an honest man of himself.

The Bishop was rightfully wronged but did something amazing. He offered his tunic and turned the other cheek. This Bishop's action changed the lives of so many in that one little moment of time. If he had not responded the way he did, Jean Valjean would be imprisoned for life. This act of grace and love was the propeller to steer change in this ex-con. The story goes on as he opens a factory, becomes mayor, and takes in an orphan. Valjean learned to extend his tunic, all because someone extended it to him first.

Myriel could have just told the police there was nothing stolen and called it a day, but he took it a step further and insisted on giving the candlesticks too. He went out of his way to promote a second chance and gave more than he should. We too can extend love and mercy to others who do not deserve it, in hopes that our moment in time could change the lives of others as well.

"The robbed that smiles, steals something from the thief."
—William Shakespeare

When in battle, we need to identify when we should stand our ground and fight, or stand down and turn the other cheek. It can be frustrating not to fight, especially if rightfully wronged. God has given us the ability to choose—free will. We have the choice to work out and the choice of which exercises to perform. We can bike rather than run. We can share Christ with others vocally, be a silent witness, or ignore the entire issue. We can be a truth teller or talebearer. We can be peacemakers or stir up gossip and strife. If I am supposed to invite someone to church but choose that "I" do not want to go out of my

 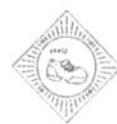

way to do this, then someone who is gifted with discipleship may not have the opportunity to use their gifts. We are all part of the equation and are all called to be the hands and feet of Jesus in our individual ways.

What would our culture be like if we all gave our cloaks, turned our cheeks, and loved our enemies? What if we went out of our way to help others instead of ignoring their issues or needs? You may not need to give candlesticks, but you could give time, love, or forgiveness. Even if we extend Christ's love and people don't accept it, we are called to be obedient.

ARMOR ALERT: Holiness

1. **Has there ever been a time when you went out of your way to show mercy and peace to someone else who did not deserve it?**

2. **Has someone else ever done this for you?**

Week 7, Day 4
A Time to Share

"But in your hearts honor Christ the Lord as holy, always being prepared to make a defense to anyone who asks you for a reason for the hope that is in you; yet do it with gentleness and respect."
—1 Peter 3:15, ESV

A few years ago there was an older lady in one of my fitness classes who came dependably three times per week for years. She was a delightful, beautiful little thing with smiles and compliments. One day during class I could tell something was very wrong with her physical body. When I asked, she said she did not have much longer to live because a disease was attacking her nervous system. I was shocked when I heard the disease took her only a few short days after. The genuine grief came when I heard she did not have a relationship with God. I thought she knew the Lord based on her daily moral living. I missed the opportunity to make sure her eternal life was secured in her faith while instructing her physical health all those years. I just assumed she knew Christ. I truly understand God is the judge and not me, and maybe there is hope she spoke with someone else before her passing, but I could have at least made sure she knew Jesus while she was here with me.

Even though someone is a good moral person, that does not mean they have a relationship with God. I was a friend, but not the faith friend I could have been. I have learned I cannot sit idle with my assumption that someone is a Jesus follower. We should pray and seize opportunities to share our faith when they arise because that moment in time might never present itself again. Even when inconveniences come our way, those instances might be part of God's larger plan. For example, if we spill coffee on our clothes on the way to work, we could be spared from a deadly crash. This simple spill may seem like a huge inconvenience, but not when we consider that God spared our life.

We are all called to go out and witness, either by word or deed (Colossians 3:17, Matthew 28:19, Acts 1:8). Verbally sharing Jesus could send frightening lightning bolts up some spines. Many people do not know what to say, do not want to impose on others, or are insecure about their own salvation. A few pages ago, you read that others cannot refute your testimony because it belongs to you personally. The Bible tells us people hear the message of the cross very clearly through our very own testimony of meeting Christ. If it is as easy as sharing an actual experience, then it takes a lot of pressure off trying to think on the spot of what to say. Do not worry if you think they will ask a question you may not be able to answer. Let them know you do not have it all together or all the answers, but that you do know Christ is the way, the truth, and the life. You can also tell them you will find out the answer to their question. Talk to a pastor or friend to find the answer and take it back to that person.

We are told in the Bible to be prepared to give an answer of the hope we have in Christ if others ask. We do not need to depend on our own strength in witnessing. Acts 1:8 reads, "And you will receive power when the Holy Spirit comes on you, and you will be My witnesses…" The Holy Spirit's power will give us the words to say. Our job is to do what He asks and be prepared to share in word or deed. Our word is our testimony, and this is something we all already know. Do not stress if you do not know what to say just yet. It does not have to be perfect either. Some may need to take a little time to have their testimony ready to share with more confidence and comfort.

Sharing the Gospel with peace is part of the Armor of God that we are all called to wear. At times I can feel the gift of evangelism rising inside of me. I can easily invite others to church, prayer meetings, and Bible studies. However, there are times I feel this gift is as far from me as Florida is from California. I sometimes do not trust the Holy Spirit and feel like it is all on me to relay the Gospel to them with perfect speech. But this is where I am learning to trust the Holy Spirit. If we feel called to say something, we should, even though the results may not end up as we anticipated. It is not we who are being rejected; it is Christ.

This Scripture helps me to defend and protect my Jesus: "Always be ready to give a defense to everyone who asks you a reason for the hope that is in you" (1 Peter 3:15). If we are engaging socially with others and they are not ready to hear what we have to say, the Bible says in Matthew 10:14 to leave the seed you planted and let another come and water or harvest it. It is not our job to control the outcome of a certain soul. God has blessed us with brothers and sisters in Christ to go out and labor together for Him.

If I do not feel led, then I do not pursue. I may have a gift or urge to share, and maybe you are the person to mentor, disciple, befriend, love, encourage, or listen. We are all a part of the body of Christ. We cannot all be the mouth. Some of us are the ears, the hands, and the feet.

ARMOR ALERT: Time to Share

Share a testimony with your AP/AG about how you met Jesus or something He proved, showed, revealed, took, gave, or allowed in your life. (Sometimes it helps to write it out and see it on paper.)

Trainer Talk

Your testimony is so very precious to our Lord Jesus. I challenge you to share it with more than just your AP. You can even write a comment on my web site and tell me the story (I would love that!). This 2-Week Relationship Challenge could be a little difficult to measure daily or even weekly, but keep moving forward with it. Pray for excellence in all you do with this challenge! It could change the way you connect with others. I know you can do this. Please talk to your AP about your challenge.

Before You Meet

Shod my Feet with the Preparation of the Gospel of Peace

Moment for Meditation

Father in heaven, show me this day how to be better and thrive in my relationships with others. Give me peace in my heart with Your love for me.

I put on the belt of truth and ask You to help me keep truth girded around me at all times. Help me to cling to the truth of the Gospel and recognize false claims.

I put on the breastplate of righteousness and ask You to help me keep my heart clean from sin. I ask for forgiveness from my poor choices. Please forgive me. Help me to not follow the "I." Protect my heart from the enemy and give me strength to cling to You at all times. Help me identify how to deal with the root of my addictions and cravings. Show me where I fall short and where I can improve. I give You my body and my mind. Fill me with Your love for other people.

I put on the Gospel of peace. Help me to identify the crazy cycles in my life and to give me wisdom on how to stop them. I ask that You take all anxiety away from my heart and fill it with peace. In the places I am lacking, fill me with love. Put kindness on my lips and abundant joy in my heart.

Show me the truth in Your Gospel message so I can share it by word or deed. Help me to be peaceful no matter where I am and what I do. Give me the courage to share my testimony with others. In Jesus' name, amen.

IT'S TIME TO MEET!

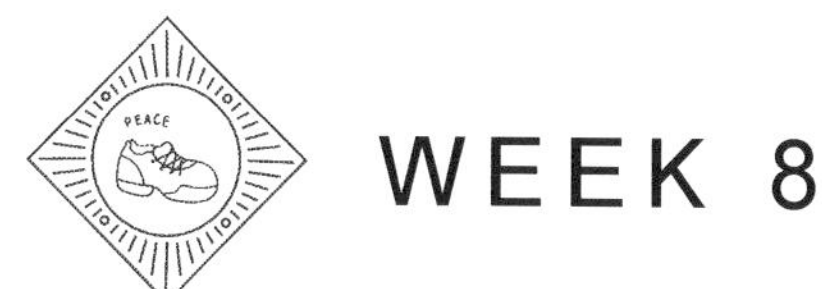

WEEK 8

ARM YOURSELF WITH SOCIAL HEALTH

Week 8, Day 1
Faith Friends

"Salt is good, but if salt has lost its taste, how shall its saltiness be restored? It is of no use either for the soil or for the manure pile."
—Luke 14:34-35a, ESV

Food that does not have flavor is not that enticing to eat, regardless of how good it looks. If I told you to eat only plain broccoli at lunch for two weeks, you would not get too excited about it. If I told you to eat broccoli, but you could add anything to it, most would accept the challenge. Anything plain is just that—plain. If the Gospel we preach is not seasoned with Christ's grace, love, and peace, it is undesirable to others. Likewise, friendships require the same seasoning.

We should seize opportunities to deepen our relationships with our faith friends and make it a point for those in the faith to bond, challenge, hold accountable, encourage, and pray together. When I am busy with my schedule, I slack in my relationships—even the ones that mean the most to me (this is why it is important to organize our desires and time). It is not that I do this on purpose, but sometimes life pulls at me, and I allow myself to retract and pull back to focus on myself. When I pull back too much, I end up straining relationships without even knowing it.

Our faith friends help promote health to our body too—when their focus is off the "I." Friends that hold similar spiritual values promote peace and love without jealousy, envy, deceit, or bitterness. These exceptional friends can be closer than our earthly family at times because they are our 'forever' spiritual family. They love us as we should be loved, without reserve, unconditional, as Christ's love flows in and through them. It is a spiritual love that will grow our relationships in a deeper way. Cling to these faith friends because they refresh, strengthen, and energize you with a willing desire to see the best in you.

In college, I had the privilege of being surrounded by many faith friends. Their relationships with me involved more than sharing dreams and secrets. Not only would I have tons of fun and fill hours with laughing, but I would also be called out for my mishaps. The reason why they were amazing was that they called me out in love and in a non-judgmental way, seeking to see me thrive instead of seeing me repeat failures. It was all to make me a better Christ-follower. My friends would tell me when I was wrong, or when I needed to improve my cleaning skills on my side of the dorm room. I respected them for it. It helped mold me into the faith friend that I am today. They promoted peace at all costs and loved me with everything that came with me—the good, bad, and ugly.

The enemy wants to kill and destroy these close-knit relationships because they are promoting Jesus in their very nature. Faith friends seek after Christ and encourage each other to continue the spiritual race set before them. When faith friends pray together, especially about conflict, God meets them and is there with them (Matthew 18:20). The very nature of our friendships are built around faith, and that faith is powerful enough to move mountains in the spiritual world (Matthew 17:20). Faith friends are not perfect. There will be times they do the opposite of what we hope (I am living proof of that). It is entirely plausible that the enemy will attack these friendships more intensely because it hurts and wounds us on a deeper level.

A simple secret can separate the best of friends, according to the Bible. This is why we must be the best faith friend we can be through God's help. If we mess up, we know to repent and seek forgiveness immediately, before the "I" gets in the way and allows elapsed time to deepen the offense. The Bible says to amend anger quickly (Ephesians 4:25). This is a tall order for sure, but something we are all capable of achieving.

One of Jesus' closest friends, Peter, turned his back on Him three times in one morning. This reiterates the invisible battle behind the scenes that the spirit world has influence on our social health—our friendships. If Peter walked with Jesus, saw and experienced miracles, and could still deny Him, I realize how much more I can screw up my relationships too. Peter learned from His faults and went on to become one of Jesus' largest megaphones, preaching the Gospel of peace wherever he went. I am convinced this spiritual conflict will continually attack our faith relationships and will strain them if we are not in daily renewal with Christ.

For Further Reading: Great examples of faith friends in the Bible include Ruth and Naomi in the book of Ruth, and David and Jonathan in 1 Samuel 18.

ARMOR ALERT: Praying For Faith Friends

Today, intentionally pray over your faith friends. Use your words from your heart. If you do not have faith friends, now is a good time to pray for them.

1. Ask God for protection, growth, joy, intimacy, love, and honor.
2. Pray against jealousy, competitiveness, and drama.
3. Ask God to bless your friendships with laughter and good memories.
4. Pray that the enemy will have no access to thwart any of your relationships.
5. Pray that you will recognize personal faults and apologize right away.

Week 8, Day 2
Flourishing or Floundering Friendships

"But the wisdom that is from above is first pure, then peaceable, gentle, willing to yield, full of mercy and good fruits, without partiality and without hypocrisy. Now the fruit of righteousness is sown in peace by those who make peace."
—James 3:17-18

Relationships come in all different shapes, sizes, colors, frequencies, and blessings. Women are particularly aware that some friendships are easy to maintain and grow, while others take varying levels of energy. People move, some take different paths, jobs can intervene, and death can separate. People come and regularly go throughout our journey on earth, but the real testament is how we invest in these friends while we are able.

Rearing friendships in high school, junior high, and elementary school with my five daughters has its learning curve. I can say I now have firsthand experience that some girls can just be flat out mean. Conversations at our house happen on a daily basis concerning the real reasons behind behaviors and attitudes of peers. Kids want to be accepted, valued, loved, and cherished. When these desires are threatened, it is natural for kids to retaliate, even against friends (may I add, this is all very similar to adult friendships). If one of my daughters gets hurt by a friend, I often find out the friend is hurting herself. My goal when rearing my girls is to teach them to help the hurting friend, instead of retaliating.

"Is any pleasure on earth as great as a circle of Christian friends by a good fire?"—C.S. Lewis

There are many reasons why friendships flounder. If we were honest, sour people could easily inhibit us from making sweet lemonade. People are life. Without others, we would die from loneliness. This is exactly why God made Adam's helper, Eve, why babies do not thrive without being held and loved, and one reason why depression hits the hearts of so many women today—they are alone, afraid, and do not feel cherished. God tells us to prepare our feet with peace. If we were truly peaceful and humble of heart, without jealousies in our relationships, we could very well change our lives and the lives of those around us.

I once said a funny remark (as sometimes a *Miss Smarty-Pants* does) in a conversation with the intent to bring a light-hearted tone to a situation. It was a few days later when someone else confronted me that my comment wasn't taken the way I intended. This was when a flourishing friendship took a turn. My apology was heartfelt as I explained the situation, but it was not accepted. The enemy was having his way with both of us, and our friendship was sinking fast. Through the months that followed, I harbored bitterness in my heart. I was deeply wounded by the whole situation. I prayed for God to help me forgive and let the pain go, but it took a very long time for it to happen fully. I realized as I walked through that low valley with friendship, how Jesus knew my pain. His friends misunderstood Him as well.

Life is so much sweeter when our social health is thriving, and it is truly the pits when it is not. We can wreck our time with other friends and family when focused on the one friendship that is strained. If you have a friendship that is floundering, Jesus is a perfect person from whom to seek intervention. He surrounded Himself with 12 good friends, had a small group of even better friends, and a smaller group of best friends. Even those close friends rejected Him at one point in their time together. In His larger group, He was loved and betrayed. In His smaller group, He was honored and deserted. Even one of His best friends rejected knowing Him three times in one pivotal morning. He knows what it feels like when a friend is anything but the best. Even though His friends wounded Him, He remained steadfast with grace and love for them. He forgave them and even gave His life in the midst of it all.

Holding on to bitterness with an unforgiving heart wounded me personally with undesired mind games, emotional distress, and a halt in a flourishing relationship. I later learned my friend had something deeper going on in her life that I didn't know. We prayed together and began to mend what was torn. We can encourage, protect, show grace, and let things go when we lace prayer with friends. I know it can be super hard to pray with some friends (it might even feel worse than public speaking), but remember, the enemy will place roadblocks in the way to try and destroy your precious relationships—especially by keeping prayer out of them. May we all be a friend that is full of forgiveness, grace, and love.

ARMOR ALERT: Relationship Evaluation

1. **Answer the few questions below about your closest friends and acquaintances.**
    a. Do they get jealous or competitive when you spend time with others?
    b. Do they lend pressure to spend more money than you want?
    c. Do they make you act one way when with them and another when apart?
    d. Do they put you down in front of others?
    e. Do they ever encourage you in front of others?
    f. Do they talk about God with you?
    g. Do they ever ask to pray for you?
    h. Do they hold grudges with you?
    i. Do they get mad at you often?
    j. Do they have the freedom to call you out on something in love without you being offended?

2. **Since this entire section is really all about *you*, the questions above are really for *you*. Turn the tables and exchange the questions to read in the first-person, and then honestly answer them.**

3. **If you have a relationship strain, pray that God would help mend it, for God to show you who your close friends are, and which ones need your attention. If you need a special friend, ask God to send that person your way and that you would recognize them when they arrive.**

Trainer Talk

Your 2-Week Relationship Challenge is underway. Pray and ask God to help if you are struggling with your social health. Insecurity, jealousy, or a number of things may be hurled at us, and make us retract in seclusion from others. Utilize this opportunity to put on the Gospel of peace. Make Him your focus. Remember, others will not like us merely because we love Jesus. Ask Him to give you ideas to fulfill your relationship challenge with surprising outcomes and to have many opportunities to enrich the lives of those around you.

Week 8, Day 3
Muzzle Thy Mouth

"A talebearer reveals secrets, but he who is of a faithful spirit conceals a matter."
—Proverbs 11:13

As the different activities and busyness of life flood our schedules, it can make for some overdrawn kids. These children can come to practice late, upset, rushed, or starving (a perfect setup for relationship drama to unfold while undergoing drills on the practice field). You bet a snarled look from this overdrawn kid is going to make its way to the eyes of teammates. Undeserved drama allows one girl to rise against the other. A thoughtless social media post after a hard practice can start an online disaster. Rumors form and gossip spreads as the "likes" and comments tally, all while the kid rushed to practice with little sleep, without a nutritious meal, and stress of tons of homework is defamed.

Gossip is like a lit match dropped on the parched ground in a wooded forest. I do not need to spell out how gossip maligns, destroys, and divides friendships. We have all seen our share of this nasty friendship rivalry. We damage our personal credibility if we merely stand by a circle of gossipers. I know a dear friend who refuses to gossip or speak poorly of others. She is not perfect but is still well known as a listening vault. She keeps matters tucked away in her heart, and no one has the key. This is someone who I admire deeply.

Whispers separate the best of friends (Proverbs 16:28). Gossip is casual or unconstrained conversation or reports about other people, typically involving details that are unconfirmed as being true.[11] You may personally not have an issue with gossip at all. Some conversations I hear are borderline gossip (which really means it is). In faith circles, I have experienced instances of people who ask for prayer over their relationships but give too many private details, all in the name of how best to pray for the situation. Asking prayer for a friend is a precious gift that should not be tossed and mixed like a salad. We need to honor our friends and keep our sharing straightforward. If we pass on a prayer request about someone else, ask God to show you which details are important and which to pray within your own heart. God is God and knows exactly what is going on anyway.

I love to talk a lot, and it has gotten me in trouble sometimes. I often pray for God to muzzle my mouth and teach me to recognize when gossip is getting ready to burst out. He indeed has answered my prayer. One summer I was shocked just how much it was around me—even though I wasn't the one spewing it this time. Groups of friends in the stands all around me were all in on it. It was like I was at a gossip festival. God opened my eyes and allowed me to hear and see this fire-breathing animal spreading destruction all around. It was then that I made the decision that I couldn't just sit there and think I wasn't a part of the situation. I was just as guilty listening, even though I was intently trying not to. Just being there was making me feel sick. I had to do something more than just getting up and leaving. I had to say something to stop it (which was also making my nauseous). God gave me the strength to

 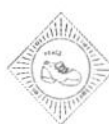

stop the conversations. I told everyone around me to look at the reason why we were here, to focus on the game. After the awkward pause, the gossip stopped. I'm sure I was the center of gossip later, but I did the right thing.

Just imagine what the world would be like if we did not air others' laundry, but instead held matters close to our hearts and in prayer. We do not know what other people are going through, so we cannot judge. Proverbs is a fabulous book filled with golden nuggets to enrich our lives. This isn't just good advice. It is God's Holy Word and which He intends us to follow. We have all heard the passage that suggests taking the plank out of our eye instead of examining the speck in our neighbor's. This is one tall order to follow because no adult I know likes to admit they have problems. It is humiliating. If I'm corrected by my husband (oh let's say for purposely repaying him the favor of not putting gas in the truck in a time crunch), I'm not following this proverb when I allow the "I" in all it's selfishness to point out his fault first. The friends I admire most are those who are humble when they accept the plank in their eyes and don't even look for the speck in their neighbor's.

I have learned by countless errors on my part that I cannot assume someone came to the same meeting as I did with a smile and hot coffee in hand. They could have just had a fight with their spouse, an argument with their teenager, or heard a bad report from the physician. Depression could be flooding their heart or jealousy ripping apart their mental health. We cannot afford to speculate and pass judgment on others.

God does not strike people down with a lightning bolt every time they sin, but that is what it feels like when gossip makes a grand entrance. When a scandal arises again, grab the opportunity to make things right. Consider defending the one dumped on or deliberately walking away to make a point. Sometimes we might not be able to stop it right there, like if we are in a packed board meeting or listening to a speaker. However, pray there are opportunities to amend the situation at a later time. This is a call for bravery and courage. To call someone out on an offense can complicate a situation. Others might not hold the same morals or not seem to care one way or another. We all know deep down that gossip hurts, regardless if in the faith or not. We all know right from wrong. Be an intentional gossip stopper and promote peace. Others will ultimately respect you in the long run.

ARMOR ALERT: In the Ring of Gossip?

1. **Do you notice gossip when it is happening?**

2. **Are you generally a spreader or the defender of gossip?**

3. **If you notice gossip in your small group of friends, or with any faith friends, take a few seconds within your heart and pray. Right now, ask the Holy Spirit to show you when it's happening next time and to help you stop it or have strength to leave the conversation.**

Week 8, Day 4
Giving the Best in Each Relationship

"For the whole law can be summed up in this one command: "Love your neighbor (friends, family members, spouse, boss, co-worker, significant other) as yourself."
—Galatians 5:14, author comments added

Time is fleeting and only available for the here and now. You cannot guarantee there will be a tomorrow or that you have time available. A wise friend told me—what you do with your time is the reflection of your heart and desires. Carving out moments to strengthen your relationships is one of the most important action steps for a healthy life. We need others to have a thriving life (that is why God created Eve for the first male). God demonstrated we should not live alone or in seclusion. Relationships are one of the most precious gifts we have. This is why the elite prisoners are given seclusion; the maximum penalty short of death—being alone.

My husband and I carved out date night at least once per week before the kids were born to make sure we connected on a deeper level. Even if we could not afford going out to dinner as often as I would have loved, we still did things together like; taking a walk or bike ride, swinging at the park, trying a new workout program, sitting on the porch, or just watching a movie at home—with air-popped corn.

Time is a huge target the enemy tries to attack when it comes to relationships. If you feel you have no time with your spouse, your kids, or your friends, you are not just busy, you are too busy; and under attack. We need specific times set aside not only to breathe and relax alone, but also to talk about important thoughts and purposes in life, and to be ourselves with others.

Even good church activities can make family time evaporate if serving too much. Time does not mean we need to give tons of it. I am referring to the genuine quality of it. We give our best moments to what is most important. If I am on my phone when my kids are around but I am still there in the room with them, they know the time given is shared. They know my focus is not on them. If I listen and take even a few moments to look them in the eyes and really hear what they are communicating, it bonds us together and creates quality time for us all.

"We give our best moments to what is most important."

Quality time comes in many different forms. Some husbands do not want to have small talk after work; they just want to be in the same room with their spouse. My oldest daughter can fill an empty space with conversation, and I welcome her for it. I am blessed to know almost everything going on in her life. However, I have friends who do not speak nearly as much, but I can still read their non-verbal communication loud and clear. If I demanded my quieter child to tell me more things, I would not be respecting her and would hinder our relationship. Each person desires to give and receive with different avenues of communication. This is what makes relationships what they are—precious and all different.

Our relationships with God and each other are the most important commandments. Life is all about relationships. Let's be honest; it may feel completely unnatural to love others when they are nasty, unloving, or do not look and act the same as us. Love is not a feeling; it is an action. We must take action and engage appropriately in our relationships with each other just as we do with God. We have to be active in them. Our relationships need constant attention and healthy substances to grow and remain strong, just like our physical bodies.

Even if we do not currently have immediate family living around us, God has blessed us with friendships. Jesus spent more quality time with his friends. Friends bring fulfillment and blessing and can make us a stronger friend in the end.

We all have areas to work on concerning our personal interactions with others. Maybe we need to hold our tongues, give more compliments, take more opportunities to pray together, or encourage and be more accountable. Sometimes we need to sacrifice in order to follow Jesus' commandments, "'Love the Lord your God with all your heart and with all your soul and with all your mind.' This is the first and greatest commandment. And the second is like it: 'Love your neighbor as yourself'" (Matthew 22:38-39). Both of these commandments require time and effort. Our friendships will require sacrifice, time, and effort too. Strive and pray so you can give the best in each precious relationship.

ARMOR ALERT: Quality Sacrifices

1. **Who in your life needs more quality time from you?** (Maybe it's more than one person?)

2. **What specific action steps are you going to take to accomplish this with excellence?** (Include how and when.)

 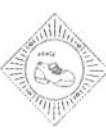

Testimony

My parents found out that I had scoliosis at six months old, severe scoliosis that required me to wear a back brace 24 hours a day, seven days a week, from six months old until age nine. At nine I had a spinal fusion and was in a body cast for months. I wore a back brace through grade school and finally by junior high I only had to sleep in it. Thank God we lived close to the best hospital around for my condition, and we had insurance. Both of my parents were active in organized sports and instilled in me the importance of having a healthy body, regardless of the handicap I faced. Being physically fit never came easy to me (and still doesn't), even though I was a starter on the varsity volleyball and basketball team through high school.

After my daughter was born when I was 35, I was the heaviest and unhealthiest I had ever been. My little girl needed a mom that could run and play and be a role model for her. So, I rejoined the gym and I enlisted with a few friends in a boot camp challenge. That challenge gave me a jump start and my energy soared. Soon after, I hired Sarah to train me in her "Buddy-Up" program. This came with more accountability and new challenges, but also a sense of being part of a team and a friendship. I continued with the group fitness classes that were offered and made new friends, both old and young, and from varying backgrounds.

I ended up running my first 5K (10-minute miles). We kept training and I turned in my personal best about a year after my first race (8:34 miles). I was with my friend Mary (age 60) when she ran her first 20-minutes without stopping, and ran her first 5K. I helped another friend, Gretchen, run her first 5K. It struck me like crazy when she told me that she looked to me as her role model. Me? No way! It was amazing as our fitness and friendship grew.

Gretchen and I worked in similar high stress and high travel jobs, and even both had employees struggling with terminal cancer. We both were juggling how to be the best wife, mom, and employee we could be. Having each other and the support of our "gym family" was critical. I will never stop training. I love the ongoing challenges. There is always more to learn and do. As for my personal strength and fitness, well, I'm still not the fastest or the strongest, but I keep trying. Sure my back bothers me, but there is more that I can do than that I can't.

Jen McCubbin
Rosemount, MN

Before You Meet

It has already been another two weeks! You should be getting comfortable with your Pre-Evaluation Chart. The focus these two weeks was on our social witness and relationships. What particular nuggets from these two chapters will you share with your AP?

Left side of chart: unfriendly, uncommitted, closed, wounded, a gossiper, a liar, a slanderer, Miss Attitude, flighty, aloof, draining on others, a manipulator, pressuring others

Right side of chart: keeper of friendships, open, loving, available, a listener, thinking of others, serving others, tender-hearted, accepting, patient, honest

Trainer Talk

Take just a few minutes to evaluate your 2-Week Relationship Challenge. Do you need to continue with the challenge or pick a new one within this challenge? Remember to shod your feet with the Gospel of peace wherever you go and whatever you do. Take God with you, in all circumstances.

Look your AP in her eyes and tell her how you appreciate how she helps you personally.

IT'S TIME TO MEET!

SECTION FIVE

SHIELD OF FAITH

No matter our beliefs in this current life, we are all on a spiritual journey with invisible spiritual forces and beings interacting on some level. We cannot see the spiritual world unfolding in every activity, but we are a spirit and are linked undeniably to this alive, unseen realm. We know deep down we have a purpose for this current time in history. With that purpose comes the drive for life itself, the propeller of our journey. Everyone has faith and spiritual cause; what varies is their level of it and where or in whom they place it.

If someone rejects Christ, his or her faith is not in Christ, but rather in something else, like an idea, another person, or another god. Some have faith in a statue and others in their wallets. Regardless if faith is attached to God, a spiritual being, a thing, or a practice, we all have a spiritual side to us linked with some kind of faith.

These next two weeks compliment each other as they present a connection between our faith and our spiritual health. Get ready to kick off your next 2-Week challenge focused on a spiritual life in Christ.

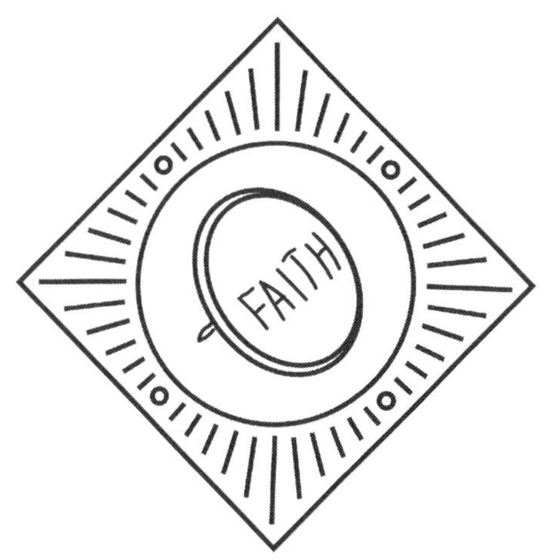

Week 9: Arm Yourself with Faith
Week 10: Arm Yourself with Spiritual Health

Health Challenge #4
2-Week Stepping out in Faith Challenge

Spiritual disciplines help us become stronger and wiser in our daily life. You may already do several of these disciplines below. Either way, choose one or two spiritual applications to focus.

1. Fasting	Give up food or sacrifice something, with focused prayer.
2. Silence	Do not speak; go to a quiet place and listen for Him.
3. Solitude	Be alone only with God.
4. Secrecy	Do not let your right hand know what your left hand is doing—perform random acts of kindness.
5. Submission	Assert yourself to come completely under the authority, wisdom, and power of Jesus.
6. Soul Befriending	Engage with others in a prayer group or speak and practice spiritual disciplines together with them.
7. Bible Reading	Search for wisdom and guidance as you study Scripture.
8. Prayer	In humility and all honestly, let your requests and heart be made known to Him.
9. Service	Have compassion on others and do something in love and outside the norm.
10. Personal Reflection	Pay attention to your inner self and seek to grow in love for God and His people.
11. Ministry	Meet the needs of other people around you in any way you feel the Holy Spirit leading you.
12. Meditation	Choose one verse only and pray and seek God about it, asking Him how to apply it to your life.
13. Discipleship	Help others around you grow in their faith and obedience to Jesus.
14. Prayer Meetings	Attend one or start one on a weekly or monthly basis.
15. Volunteer	Help in a new way, using your gifts to glorify God.
16. Following	Practice asking the Holy Spirit to lead you, then obey and follow.

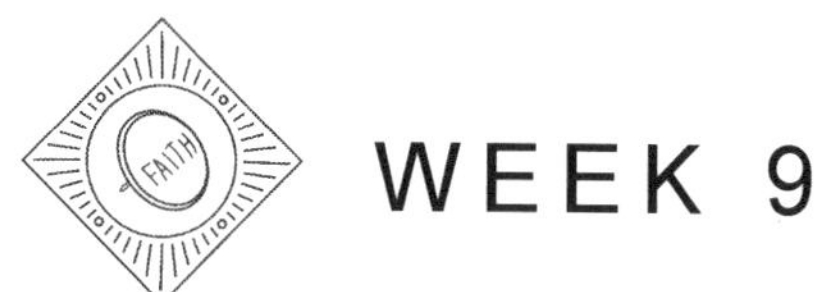

WEEK 9

ARM YOURSELF WITH FAITH

Week 9, Day 1
Shield of Faith

"Above all, taking the shield of faith with which you will be able
to quench all the fiery darts of the wicked one."
—Ephesians 6:16

A shield protects. A soldier without a shield is like an infant without sunblock at the Florida summer pool. When not protected correctly, the outcome could be fatal. We do not go into a war unless we are armed and shielded with protection—and have a cause for the encounter. Faith creates momentum for action and drives us spiritually. Faith without works is dead according to the Bible (James 2:20). When we fight on behalf of our country, we fight for freedom, safety, and justice, and have faith in our cause. Think about if there was no reason to fight. Without faith there is no hope, without hope there is death. Hope is what makes us jump out of bed in the morning and what drives our passions in life. "Faith is the substance of things hoped for and the evidence of things unseen" (Hebrews 11:1). We cannot see the driving force of faith, but it is there, just like the sun that can torch an infant's delicate skin. The sunburn demonstrates the evidence of the invisible rays of the sun. The spiritual world demonstrates evidence even though it is unseen as well. We too cannot always see the enemy coming, which is why we need to be ready and protected, with shields raised, so he cannot pierce our hearts.

Physical death is just a part of this life. Our physical body expires one day. If there were no hope for anything after death, our lives would be the hugest waste of time after our mere average of 85 years on this earth. Life would ultimately be pointless. Some believe we gain all this knowledge and hold on to experiences from this world only for them to lie wasted in the grave while we just sleep eternity away and keep dreaming, or be erased and reincarnated into something else. It does not make sense to be created with a soul if only to relinquish it after our time on earth without a purpose for remembering.

Life does go on after this life; it is just not here on this earth in the same context. Of all the spiritual leaders of this world, none spoke more about the afterlife and proved it by experiencing it, than Jesus. He is proof there is more than just the here and now and more than just a grave awaiting our death.

"Without faith it is impossible to please God" (Hebrews 11:6). If we have no faith in God, then we are doing everything in vain and are pleasing ourselves, the "I." We can serve in the soup kitchen and give all our money to the poor, but it will not please God if our hearts are not doing it for Him, even though it may secretly make us feel good. Our good deeds will not make any difference except to the "I," momentarily anyway. Spiritual matters have nothing to do with material service or gain of personal satisfactions. All throughout the Bible, God demonstrated His miraculous glory when people placed faith in Him. Hebrews 11 tells of remarkable historical events of His people who laid down everything for their faith in God. His followers did more than amazing things because there was motivation behind their will.

Our spiritual health is the most important component of health. Almost everyone will call out to God with his or her last breath or in times of urgency. When things are out of our hands, we ultimately seek divine help. We inherently know there is a higher power and someone who created the intricacies that we cannot comprehend. The Bible says our spirit will transfer to a heavenly body—for those who are a new creation in Christ (more reading of this transformation in Isaiah 65:17-18 and 2 Corinthians 5:1-10). Our spiritual health is what we have when there is nothing left in the present. It is what becomes the most important aspect when lying hopelessly in a hospital bed. Not all people will be physically healthy and able to prolong their lives by eating well and exercising. Disease will claim some who are not ready to leave, just as a car accident can call someone home too early for our standards. No matter when our time is up, our spiritual souls will have no time left to regroup. Our preparation time is at hand. The clock is ticking, whether we pushed start or not.

A shield is not just for protection. It is also a weapon. Having faith in God's Word is our shield to stave off the devil. Jesus had complete faith in God and used that faith with authority to repel the enemy. Satan twisted Scripture, trying to deceive, but Jesus replied with the truth of the living Word. God's Word has supernatural authority that the enemy is under, and silences him. The way to use the shield of faith is to use Scripture actively. If an attack comes to our mind, we can shield ourselves from it just as Jesus did when He was tempted in the wilderness. He used Scripture. We can also renew our minds daily by asking the Holy Spirit to help. This way, we can recognize the wolf in sheep's clothing and be able to uncover the enemy's tricks, schemes, and plans.

If we have faith in the Bible and believe the truth in them, there is purpose in our battles—there is purpose in our living. We are not just living to live or fighting to fight. There is a reason behind everything we do and say. If we do not know what the Scriptures say, how will we be able to use them against our enemies?

Those who do not know or have faith in Christ are unprotected from spiritual forces, and whatever shield they currently use is of no effect. It is like paper wafting in the wind. The fiery darts of Satan will be able to catch that paper shield on fire faster than they could call 911. God is not fire insurance. He is beyond a safe stairwell to heaven. He created heaven with His Word and is preparing a place for those who love Him in truth.

ARMOR ALERT: Faith Recap

"Who through faith are shielded by God's power until the coming of the salvation that is ready to be revealed in the last time" (1 Peter 1:5).

We do not go to church just to feel good and earn attendance "brownie points" with God—and congregation members. The church is for us to glorify God, discipleship, and bond together in love with other believers—the two greatest commandments. Think about your honest motivation for attending church. Assuming you were able to go to church this week, take a moment to recap the sermon. Do not go to the next question without genuinely answering each question below in your heart.

1. **Did God speak to your heart while in the service?**
2. **Was there conviction or jubilation inside of you?**
3. **Was your faith in God built-up while listening to the sermon?**
4. **Did you worship with a pure heart or with a facade and out of duty?**
5. **Did you include, challenge, or encourage other people while there?**
6. **Did your conversations have anything to do with God before or after the service when talking to other people?**
7. **What is one thing you learned from the service?**

Week 9, Day 2
The Crossing Spirit World

"Above all, taking the shield of faith with which you will be able to quench all the fiery darts of the wicked one."
—Ephesians 6:16

The smart and conniving devil wants us to fail at everything we do. He is here to steal, kill, and destroy (John 10:10). This is why it is so important to be rooted and anchored in the truth of the Bible. If we know little about how to defend the Bible and its truths, and even less about the spirit world, we fall prey to Satan's attacks. We believe our battles are from someone else, bad luck, or karma, and do not attribute them to whom they belong. If we blame the woes of this world on other humans, it seems easy enough to move on and not worry about those invisible spiritual forces of evil. There is a theme of spiritual activity throughout the entire Bible. 1 Timothy 4 tells of this activity at all times, even our current time in history. It tells us to depart from evil for true spiritual health.

To depart from evil, our first step is to become closer to God. You should see a theme throughout this book. Everything comes back to God's Word and prayer. These are not the only two ways to connect with Christ and depart from evil, however. Spiritual disciplines will also pull you closer to Christ and take the focus off the "I"—this is what your 2-Week Challenge is dedicated to. When we are filled with God, we are not filled with other things.

The Bible teaches that spiritual warring is not limited to the unseen world. According to Hebrews 13:2, some of us entertain angels and we do not even know it. I have heard many firsthand experiences of people who have seen angels. The Bible explicitly forbids that we attempt contact with spirits that pretend to be spirits of the dead—familiar spirits. Deuteronomy 18:11 reads, "There shall not be found among you...anyone who practices divination or tells fortunes or interprets omens, or a sorcerer or a charmer or a medium or a necromancer or one who inquires of the dead, for whoever does these things is an abomination to the Lord." These things seem to be intriguing to some, but they are all from Satan and his demons. They are here to trick and deceive us.

The Bible states that dead people do not have contact with the living (Luke 16:19-31). If someone has contact with or experiences a spiritual being that says they are from the dead, you can be sure it is not Great-Grandpa. Rather, it is a spirit pretending to be him. This is why we are warned to not interact with those who claim to contact the dead. We are contacting fallen angels, unclean spirits, and demons. They may come to us in a calming way, luring us to believe they are our friends or from God. They may appear to be nice, forthcoming in their appearance and communication, but they are deceitful spirits under the control of the father of lies.

Our modern television stations believe it is perfectly fine to mess with the spirit world, interact with ghosts or spirits, and report to us they are harmless. Society is entertained as more horror movies are created. My soul was burdened as a young teenager when I watched a horror film—and I only watched glimpses of it.

2 Kings 19 tells the story of how the Lord fought a physical battle on behalf of His people. They were ready to fight, took up weapons, and put on their body armor to protect their physical bodies. In this battle, however, they did not have to use any of it. An angel of the Lord went before Jerusalem's army and snuffed the life out of their enemy. How is that for a battle plan? An important point is they did not sit on their hands, unconditioned, unmotivated, or physically wasted before a battle. No sound, earthly battle prep goes this way either. God's people still prepared their physical bodies and hearts for battle. An example to us that we still need to eat right, condition, and prepare our mental, spiritual, and emotional states to enter our battles, no matter if we physically fight in them or not.

God's awesome supernatural fighting advantage is not limited to this single example. Acts 19 and Matthew 8 report demons coming out of people in the name of Jesus and handkerchiefs that merely touched Paul's skin being taken to heal the sick—and they recovered. A demon came out of a mute and blind man because believers told it to come out in Jesus' name. While Jesus was walking this earth, He healed a naked, possessed man and returned him to his right mind because He commanded the spirits to leave. Evil spirits fear God. The enemy seems to have a lot of power, but God is the most powerful of all. Satan's demons obey Jesus when commanded because they know Jesus has ultimate authority and is ultimately the Victor on both sides of the war, as stated in Mark 1:34.

Another familiar battle is Joshua and the city of Jericho (Joshua chapter 6). After obeying God's instructions for pre-battle, the Israelites watched as God knocked down the stone walls with the willing blasts of soldiers' physical trumpets. The soldiers still had to prepare for battle, go to battle, engage in battle, and fight their enemy with the sword to finish the job after the walls came down. These steps were real and still had personal responsibility attached to them. They could not completely take themselves out of the battle because God's plan was to make them a part of fulfilling that miracle.

If we always cleaned up after our children, they would not learn to do it by themselves. We can tell them to do it, but if we never force them to clean up, we would raise up reckless adults. The same applies to us. If God, the vending machine, presented us with a miracle every time we called, we would not be any stronger than the day we came out of the womb. There are times He will go before us, and other times we will need to prepare and actually engage in a battle.

"If God, the vending machine, presented us with a miracle every time we called, we would not be any stronger than the day we came out of the womb."

I believe in miracles, but we cannot expect to wake up one morning and find our body fat went down 50 percent while we slept because we prayed for it. I do believe He can do this if He wanted. However, we helped get to our current body size. Natural steps need to be taken to make us stronger adults.

Some of these verses we have read depict fearful spiritual stories, yet they should be the most freeing of all if on Jesus' side because He is the One with ultimate authority. This same spiritual fighting (the Holy Spirit) is in those who believe in Jesus as their personal Savior—their Anchor in life. Because of Him, we can conquer anything that stands up against us that is evil. That should give us Holy Spirit goose bumps. It should illuminate something inside of our hearts and make us excited! We are more than conquerors through Christ who loves us (Romans 8:37), and we can do all things through Christ who gives us strength (Philippians 4:13).

My pastor has frequently said, "My idea of God might be different than yours, but no one has ever been saved by their *idea* of God." Just because we do not want to believe in all or some of this spirit talk does not mean it is not real. Spiritual wars are raging, and we are in the middle of it. As a Christ follower, you are the temple of the Living God and the Holy Spirit resides in you, not the devil. The devil can lead us astray to delve in temptation, but he cannot make you. Do not be scared of the enemy—the Lord of Lords is with you. Stand on His promises.

ARMOR ALERT: Spiritual Matters

1. **Are you scared, intimidated, confident, or do you have a conquering attitude about the spirit world—explain?**

2. **Do you honestly believe in your heart that God can do anything—even supernaturally beyond your thinking?**

3. **Do the Scriptures you just read make you see God more spiritually powerful than before—why?**

Trainer Talk

How is your 2-Week Stepping Out in Faith Challenge going so far? I encourage you to put forth great effort with this. Spiritual disciplines are a little different versus a common challenge. It's hard to place a checkmark once you accomplish them. Think of a bank account that increases in value over time. Compare this to your health. Over time our perspectives grow in maturity. Ask God for boldness to step out in faith and make Him first in all you do.

Week 9, Day 3
Divine Communication

"If my people, who are called by my name, will humble themselves and pray and seek my face and turn from their wicked ways, then I will hear from heaven, and I will forgive their sin and will heal their land."
—2 Chronicles 7:14

The words "prayer meeting" can make some people sweat and feel uneasy instantaneously. I know this to be the case as I have experienced it personally. When I was younger, I did not realize the special connection or the power of prayer. I knew my parents did it and knew I was supposed to as well. I knew it was a way to communicate with God, and that I sometimes did not want to. My impression was that prayer meetings were boring and I felt like I never got anything from them. As an emerging teenager, I accepted the norm that prayer was hard to be excited about because it did not always turn out how I wanted. It was not until college that everything changed.

"We believe the sun is in the sky at midday in summer not because we can clearly see the sun (in fact, we cannot) but because we can see everything else."—C.S. Lewis

We cannot see God, the Light, but by and in the Light we can see everything else. This clearly was the case in college concerning prayer. Prayer meetings were the norm at my Christ-centered University—Oral Roberts in Tulsa, Oklahoma. We were required to attend chapel services two times per week and group devotionals once a week in our dorms. There were other times of prayer—before classes, in the hallways, in small clusters in the prayer gardens, and voluntary prayer meetings before campus church on Sunday evenings. I did not have to look far to see people engaged in prayer at any time, all over campus. College kids by the hundreds were involved in prayer, and it was as if they liked it. I even thought some were addicted to it.

As an incoming freshman, I thought I knew how to pray, but soon learned I was missing it. It certainly is not hard to pray. I was just not humble, patient, or open to the answers God gave. I would get mad about not receiving my answers, my way. Testimonies were all around me, given daily on how God miraculously opened a door when one seemed forever closed. It was inspiring, refreshing, and exciting. These college kids were hooked because God was meeting their needs with emotional, mental, spiritual, physical, and social blessings. It wasn't always because He answered their prayers as they wanted, it was the relationship with Him they coveted. I not only learned how to pray, I learned why.

Prayer meetings at most churches are historically one of the lowest attended gatherings (unless after a major catastrophe). Not because we think prayer does not work or that it is unnecessary, there is something else in the invisible world pulling at people to not go. Prayer is a means by which we engage in spiritual communication with the living God. Our spirits are open to the Lord, who communicates deep within our inner soul and spirit. In a prayer meeting, this communication happens in a group setting (fearful to many). This connection strengthens a spiritual relationship. It can be a fearful thing to be that close with God, which is why some do not think they can go there. I know this all too well because the conviction of my sin was pulling me away from wanting to go to any prayer meetings when I was growing up. It was not until I sought a relationship with Christ on a continual growing basis that I learned not just how to pray, but why.

Many factors inhibit running toward a prayer meeting. It is hard to engage in public prayer when we are not in the practice of praying alone to God—in solitude. Jesus demonstrated solitude a few times in the Scriptures to connect with the Father (Luke 4, 5:16; Mark 1:35). We are to follow Jesus' example. This is a great spiritual discipline.

I've noticed there is a misconception that people think others judge them in a group prayer meeting. This is a tactic from the enemy to get us not to go. He aims fiery darts of insecurity, belittlement, pride, and fear. Fear can immobilize and make anyone stay far away. These flaming arrows instantaneously catch fire in our minds and consume us in a matter of seconds. Ask God to quench those darts. Ask God to give you a specific Scripture to combat the enemy.

The more time we spend with someone else we like, the more we want to please them, do things for them, bless them, and respect them. If we only requested things from a spouse, the "I" would be the focus. However, when I pour my love into my husband, he reciprocates. When I am honest and open with my heart, it connects us on a deeper level. The Bible says in James 4:8 that the more we draw near to God, the more He will draw near to us. He is into relationships. He created us to fellowship with Him. He created us to love Him, spend time with Him, and commune with Him. One way we do this is through prayer.

ARMOR ALERT: Spiritual Action

Take the rest of your time scheduled to work on this book, and just pray. If you are unsure of what to pray, use the Lord's Prayer that Jesus modeled for us in Matthew 6:9-13.

Week 9, Day 4
Be Refreshed and Filled

"But the Helper, the Holy Spirit, whom the Father will send in My name, He will teach you all things, and bring to your remembrance all things that I said to you."
—John 14:26

Do you ever feel like God should have created mothers with four hands instead of two? I often felt this way as I sat looking at my infant twins. People would ask how I managed with the other children while I nursed two babies, but all I could think about was how a mother of triplets survived. We all could use help, regardless if we have children or not, but sometimes it's hard to ask for it. We want to be strong and take care of everything ourselves. When I am humble enough and allow the Holy Spirit to help me, it's as if the floodgates of peace open within my spirit. My faith builds as I experience His purpose within me. Then I wonder, why I waited to ask for help and what stopped me from asking in the first place? Help can come in many forms and doesn't prove we are weak, but that we are wise.

John 16:5-15 is one of the greatest passages about the Holy Spirit in the Bible. In these verses, Jesus had just finished communicating to His disciples that things were going to be rough when He departed and that people would hate them because of Him. He comforts them, telling them it is to their advantage that He leaves because He is going to send the Helper.

The Holy Spirit knows us in our weakness (Romans 8:26) and helps us do things that we cannot do on our own strength. This should fill us with peace and give us a refreshing breath of air. Jesus was filled with the Spirit (Luke 4:1-2) to empower His path set before Him. Jesus was not only combating physical hunger during the famous 40 days in the wilderness, but He was also battling the enemy. He was defending Himself through the power of the Holy Spirit against the fiery darts. Jesus was triumphant over the entire journey as He demonstrated His "food" was to do the will of His Father (John 4:34).

Acts 1:8 reports that we will receive power when the Holy Spirit comes on us, and we will be witnesses in all the earth. Jesus demonstrated to the whole earth that He was more than an earthly King. To be tempted by the enemy and go without food for 40 days, all without sinning once is beyond holy. He was filled with something else besides food, something stronger and life sustaining—the Holy Spirit.

Every person is given the Holy Spirit as a gift the moment they accept Christ. The difference is that some allow the Holy Spirit to fill them while others never ask for help. We need the Helper to extinguish the plans of the enemy and propel us forward in our battles. We cannot *harness* the power of the Holy Spirit to use or abuse God. We can only experience this power when we surrender and humble ourselves fully to Him and as He wills (Galatians 5:25; Romans

8:4). This power is not just for our pastors and those with special evangelistic gifts; rather, it is available to every believer who willingly surrenders in submission and obedience to Him.

Our Helper, the Holy Spirit, reveals the truth of the Gospel (John 15:26-27) and gives us fruit in our lives. He guides us to witness and bring glory to God. Who we will marry, where we will live, and where we will study the Bible and go to church (2 Timothy 3:16-17) are all directives the Holy Spirit will give us. The Holy Spirit helps us put on the helmet of salvation when we do not understand Scripture. He guides us on how to apply it in combat (John 14:26; Romans 8:14; 1 Corinthians 2:6-14). He is with us in battle and in times of need as our Helper and Comforter.

I was learning to listen to the Holy Spirit a few summers ago and felt I had to write a letter to a friend. I was not sure what to write, and I was not in a close relationship with her particularly, but I felt this overwhelming urge to write a letter that very hour. I sat down and penned whatever came to me. It was a Holy Spirit-inspired letter because when I was done, I reread it and I was not sure what it meant. All I could tell was that it was an encouragement letter. I immediately placed it at her door without her knowing. Time passed, and I did not think much of it. I later found out she was thinking of quitting something very important and was waiting on God for direction. The timing was more than amazing. I had no idea what was going on or what I was speaking into her life. I was simply obedient on the timing. This Holy Spirit confirmation was what she was fervently praying for, regardless of what the answer was.

The power inside believers is a mighty supernatural force. Scripture teaches He releases His power to us when we are in submission to Him in three different ways. One is the fruit of the Spirit. Only through God's power can we exhibit love, joy, peace, patience, goodness, kindness, faithfulness, gentleness, and self-control (Galatians 5:22). I know if I did not have the Holy Spirit directing my spirit, I would not be so gentle in certain situations.

The second way the Holy Spirit releases His power in us is through witnessing to others. Scripture always refers to the power of the Holy Spirit in relationship to witnessing the glory of God (Acts 4:31), but only through His power are we able to carry this out. I have shared the Gospel a few times to others, knowing it was the Holy Spirit directing my steps. There's no way I would have been able to manufacture the particular outcomes on my own. A new believer receiving Christ for the first time is very fulfilling for me to see. It is refreshing and unexplainable.

Third, the Holy Spirit's power demonstrates through our daily living. Wherever God calls us, He will equip us with power (Zechariah 4:6), so we can do all we are called to do in His might, not our own strength. We shouldn't feel like we need to have all the answers or know the entire plan A-Z. The pressure is off. We can rest without worry when we daily connect and ask for help from the Holy Spirit.

The Holy Spirit is the driving force of power behind the Armor of God. We can put on the armor in vain and render it useless in our strength. In Ephesians 6:18, faith is the last piece of armor listed, but the last application in this section is to apply it in prayer. Prayer is the biggest aspect of having the armor and putting it on to begin with. He tells us to let our requests be made known to Him always, with all prayer and supplication in the Spirit. We arm ourselves with the Armor of God and fight this war through prayer. If we battle in prayer, then we must make sure we are in submission and obedience to the Holy Spirit in our lives, and not the work of the "I." We cannot fake it and make it in the spirit. Call on Him and ask for His help. He will fill you and refresh you.

ARMOR ALERT: Cleave to God

Ask the Holy Spirit to fill you so you can do everything in and through His power and authority. Read these Scriptures and pray them to God out of your heart.

1. **Arm Yourself Physically: Never stop learning**. "Never stop meditating on these teachings. You must think about them night and day so that you will faithfully do what is in them. Only then will you prosper and succeed" (Joshua 1:8).

2. **Arm Yourself Emotionally: Rest and be refreshed in Christ.** "If anyone thirsts, let him come to Me and drink. He who believes in Me, as the Scripture has said, out of his heart will flow rivers of living water" (John 7:37b-38).

3. **Arm Yourself Socially: Do no go in situations alone and unarmed, but seek the comfort and wisdom of others.** "A friend loves at all times" (Proverbs 17:17).

4. **Arm Yourself Spiritually: Trust in His unfailing Scripture.** "I tell you, if anyone believes in Me, he will do the things that I do; and greater things he will do, because I go to the Father" (John 14:12).

5. **Arm Yourself Mentally: Memorize and read as much Scripture as you can to help in future spiritual battles.** "So then faith comes by hearing, and hearing by the Word of God," (Romans 10:17).

Trainer Talk

The end of the week is here, and that means your 2-Week Challenge is halfway through. This challenge check-in should reminder you to keep moving forward in it. Remember, this is a challenge, so it is not always going to be easy. I'm so very proud of you. Hang in there and continue with strength.

Before You Meet
Take the Shield of Faith

Moment for Meditation

Lord God, You are mighty and righteous in all Your ways. Thank You for saving me from sin and eternal separation from You.

I put on the belt of truth today. Gird truth around my waist. Keep it tightly secured so I never lose it. Protect me from false truths of the enemy.

I put on the breastplate of righteousness and ask Your protection over my emotions and my character. Please forgive me for my sins and give me strength when I am weak. Help me to make the best decisions.

I shod my feet with the preparation of the Gospel of peace. Please fill all my relationships with joy, peace, patience, and love by taking out competition, jealousy, and negativity. I ask that You would help me recognize my failures and hang-ups in my relationships and give me wisdom and strength to fix them. Open my eyes so I can see how to be a better friend. Help me, so I am not floundering, but flourishing in each of my divinely appointed friendships.

I take the shield of faith and use it to quench the fiery darts of the enemy. Help me never to put it down and always cling to the truths and the faith I have in Jesus Christ. Help me to be an incredible warrior for You.

In the name of Jesus, amen.

IT'S TIME TO MEET!

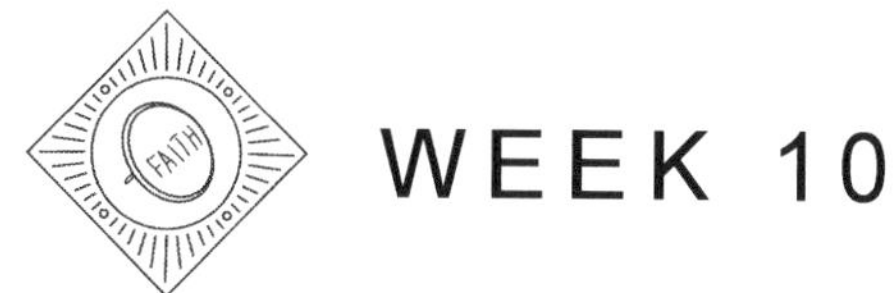

WEEK 10

ARM YOURSELF WITH SPIRITUAL HEALTH

Week 10, Day 1
The Idol

"O God, You are more awesome than Your holy places. The God of Israel is He who gives strength and power to His people. Blessed be God!"
—Psalm 68:35

An idol is anything more important, that we cling to first, or that we value more highly than God. When I hear the word idol, I think of carved structures and statues. But if an idol is anything that sets itself up higher or more important than God, that would include money, television, technology, news, politicians, bosses and CEO's, gossip, food, clothes, shopping, relationships, statuses, and the list could go on. It is plausible we all have some idol lingering around our hearts.

I used to yearn for sweets, frequently. When I knew I could not have it, I thought about it all the more. I wanted that sugary treat after dinner especially. It was calling my name from the kitchen cupboard. It was a haunting desire for something I thought I needed to make me feel better and satisfy something I was missing. This made me develop a desire for desserts after lunch too. *What's just another small piece going to harm?* It was not just the issue of consuming extra calories; the cravings were controlling my thoughts. Treats are not idols in themselves, but they can be when they control us. Just reading about delicious sweet and delectable desserts can make us want to eat some. Compare this with trashy novels and watching inappropriate movies or horror films. This fills our minds with unholy things and takes our focus off God. These provide a foothold for the enemy, who helps us think of these poor choices all the more. These poor choices, if repeated, begin to take root where good things once trumped.

Some of us have deep addiction roots. Food or drink might not be the issue behind your idol; maybe it is a dream about a knight in shining armor as you long for someone other than your spouse. It could be an addiction to social media or technology. Many addictive behaviors turn into idols. Idols consume our time and our finances, take us away from family and can desensitize us from reality. These things in themselves are not evil, but the love of them is.

When you wake up in the morning, what is one of the first things you do? Does the answer have God in it somewhere—even a good morning greeting? To include God in your morning routine, it takes time, thought, and practice. Our time with God does not have a required amount of frame, and it does not always have to be quiet and while sitting down in the morning. We can take God with us. We can spend time with Him in the transit to our job or school. We can pray in our hearts no matter where we are. If we always wait until the end of the day to meet up with God, think of all the opportunities we could have missed by not communicating and going with His ideas and plans first. Do you ever log in hours on social media without even thinking about God? We are told to be watchful, to not be taken captive by things of this world, which will pull us farther from God. Departing from evil makes our spirit at peace and brings physical health to our bones.

Spending hours with something or someone builds a deeper connection. This is why the Bible compares us to sheep. We can wander aimlessly in no time flat. We need to be reminded not to stray from the path (our callings and goals in life). We need to set goals and timelines, set markers, make signs, be accountable, and look for the finish line. If we never did these things we would forget in the middle of the race why we were running—and head down the wrong path.

I have a notebook with a lot of prayers and special moments recorded in it. There are so many prayers answered in ways I had never expected. When I prayed for something I would write the date. Sometimes I just gave the request to God and never even followed up. Once I prayed and that was the end of it. I knew it was all up to God on the outcome. But, by recording it all, I was able to see how many prayers God answered and how He answered them, many of which were not answered how I expected. If I had not written them down, I would not have remembered most of them, and I would not have been able to see how clearly He answered them.

In ancient Bible times, altars were mainly built as a monument to remember or commemorate a divine occurrence, which took place at certain locations. In Hebrew, an altar means "to slaughter" or "place of sacrifice." However, altars were also made for such things as worship, a memorial, to make a covenant, or to find refuge. All altars point to something. Noah built the first altar recorded (Genesis 8:20) and many prominent people after that made an altar at some point in the Bible. No altars are recorded in the New Testament—Jesus is our living altar (Hebrews 13:10).

During Bible times, there were thousands of places to worship, but they didn't all point toward God. Even those who were followers of satanic idols had places of worship (2 Kings 23:15). It's our very nature to worship something. Almost everywhere someone would go in ancient times; it would remind them of their spiritual purpose in life. The same is true in today's age—we have churches sprinkled throughout our cities. Think what it would look like if all the churches were gone. We need these as beacons in our lives. Think about why God created physical places to gather and worship. It was a meeting place where they could commune with God and remember His covenant. It was a memorial every time they saw it.

God is amazing because He knows we need reminders, accountability, and memorials in our lives. He knows we are human and forget. You see, we are like sheep—wandering, repeating mistakes, and going back to the same sins. We need a Shepherd and a Helper to remind us to obey and stay on the path. Pagans made altars to their gods. God ordered His people to destroy them (Exodus 23:24; Deuteronomy 12:1-3). We need to take down any idol that is distracting and taking our focus off God.

ARMOR ALERT: Idol Reflection

Answer these questions in your heart and pray for your answers.

1. **When was the last time you recorded prayers or special God moments in a journal?**

2. **If you don't record things, would you challenge yourself to start today?**

3. **Is there anything you need to take off your *altar* to replace it with God?**

Week 10, Day 2
Race of a Life Time

"But from there, you will seek the Lord your God, and you will find Him
if you seek Him with all your heart and with all your soul."
—Deuteronomy 4:29

What prize and ultimate fulfillment do you honestly strive for? This is a loaded question because there is no context attached. It would be a much different answer if I asked more specifically such as fulfillment relating to your job, relationships, goals in life, or personal leadership. It would add clarity if I also added a time frame—6 months, 10 years, or at the end of your life. We are going to dig in and read about the rewards we should strive for. There are many blessings we receive in life. Some blessings are physical in nature, some emotional, and some spiritual. When we exercise hard and try to attain a physical goal, we expect some compensation at the end—a healthier body, for example. The reason for our strivings should be the focus, but we cannot neglect the journey, the race, and the means by which we arrive.

Our earthly life is compared to a race in Hebrews 12:1-29. It is the most exciting race of all time. For some, it could be short and sweet like a sprint or treacherous and exhausting like a marathon, and of course, many places in between. During our race, we can run or jump ahead, become discouraged and lag behind, carry others when they need help, or end being carried by others. Either way, there is a finish line waiting for us, one that will be more amazing to cross than any earthly prize could offer.

In 1 Timothy chapter 6, we read an encouragement from Paul, a seasoned Christ-follower, to young Timothy in his specific role God called him to. Paul is a fantastic mentor and leads by example on running his life race for Christ with purpose and excellence. He reminds Timothy of his calling and to stand firm in it. Many of us do not know what we are striving for. We could be looking ahead barely far enough to see the next calendar month flip. Others might have their whole life planned out. But what if our strivings and goals are all amiss? Paul knew he was to travel and preach the Gospel wherever the Holy Spirit led him. Timothy was to rear up a young church in Berea. They each had specific, and different, callings and tasks set before them, but they both were striving for the same prize.

When I prepare for races, there are many different training approaches for each course. Adventure racing training is much different compared to running a marathon. The type of training also depends on how long the adventure race is and what type of temperature and terrain I will encounter. If it is a sprint of three to five miles, it necessitates much less preparation training than a 25-mile adventure race. When I sign up for a race, I have a general idea of what to expect, especially if I have run something similar in the past. However, I will never truly know the exact outcome with the different competitors, temperatures, and locations. This is the exciting part of signing up for a race.

Once we have been running a road race for a while, we can relax and focus on a steady pace. Our life race, however, is an absolute adventure with needed times of different paces. There is always something new to experience when following the Holy Spirit, just like birthing children. We have an idea of what to expect, but every delivery is different from the others. It is still an exciting yet fearful experience at the same time. We can go through childbirth because the long and painful journey was worth our bundle of blessing.

God created this earth and all that is in it. Ponder what life truly is with Him as the leader of your daily living. This race in life can be embraced with all the wonderful experiences and blessings if we truly give it to the Creator of the universe. Think if we all kept our eyes on the prize of eternity with Jesus—the Finisher of our faith (Philippians 3:14). This world would be a piece of heaven. Jesus finished His race on the cross with complete excellence and holiness even in His weakened physical body. We must ask the Holy Spirit to give us strength when we are weak (and want to throw in the towel on our nutritional goals). Embrace the help of the Holy Spirit in your life race—the calling and path God has planned for you. Ask Him to fill you daily. Ask Him to guide you, comfort you, teach you, and train you in righteousness so you can cross your next finish line with excellence.

ARMOR ALERT: Running Hard or Hardly Running?

1. **Write down your accomplishments and reflections from this week—physical, emotional, social, spiritual, or mental.**

2. **How well do you think you are striving and running in your life race? Rate yourself 1 to 10 for each health area, 10 being highest.** (Progress is the focus, not perfection.)

_____ PHYSICAL HEALTH
_____ EMOTIONAL HEALTH
_____ SOCIAL HEALTH
_____ SPIRITUAL HEALTH
_____ MENTAL HEALTH

Trainer Talk

At this point in your journey, another 2-Week challenge may seem repetitive. Ask God to revive your heart through His spiritual disciplines and for a renewed purpose and reasoning behind them. Your 2-Week Challenge should include prayer. If it doesn't, please don't skip this important meeting with God. It's not wasted time. Embrace any moment you have with Him.

Week 10, Day 3
What are You Multiplying?

"Let him know that he who turns a sinner from the error of his way will save a soul from death and cover a multitude of sins."
—James 5:20

Witnessing can come in many forms. Praying with someone to receive Christ is a blessed experience, but many times we speak the truth and leave seeds of faith, to be matured and cared for by others to harvest. I wish we could see all the fruit of our labor, but we won't always get that chance. We have to trust God in all that we do and rest in His eternal purposes.

One late summer evening a few years ago, I had the privilege of leading a young lady to Christ. She called me up in tears, weeping over some hardships, and asked if she could come over even though it was past my bedtime. She came over in a matter of minutes with open arms and hugged me for a long time. I was not on her speed dial or her top 10 frequent hangout homes, yet she knew I loved Jesus by our conversations in the community. We talked for a few hours about her life and how God was supposed to be in control of it and not the "I." She was living a life of recklessness. She knew some stories of Christ but never had a relationship with Him. She did not know she needed to have a relationship with Him. She said there was a hole in her life that she could not figure out how to fill in the right way, and she felt as if the hole was only getting deeper.

She had attended church in the past, but she never actually heard the salvation message the way she heard it that warm night in my backyard. I told her the non-sugar coated version—that she must turn away from her current lifestyle, talk to Jesus, and accept what He accomplished on the cross. After asking her if she really desired for Jesus to fill her and honestly wanted to turn from her lifestyle, she yelled at me with a loud "YES!" I have never heard anyone express with so much fervency their willingness to be saved so badly. It was a huge blessing for both of us. I got her a Bible, she started a Bible study, and the rest is HIStory.

The Holy Spirit led her to my front stoop, and prepped my mouth with words I needed to say at that moment. His timing usually is not mine. From early runs to late night talks, God can use us at any time. As comfortable as it is to read about these testimonies, it is another thing to go through them. If we are too busy to plug in daily with Christ, we could miss some of the most rewarding surprises. 1 Peter 3:15 says, "Sanctify the Lord God in our hearts and always be ready to give a defense to everyone who asks you a reason for the hope that is in you, with meekness (Gospel of peace) and fear" (author addition).

Sometimes I can be reluctant to follow that still small voice of the Holy Spirit. It is because of that recurring "I" right in the middle of the word pride. I have learned if I do ignore it, I will regret it later. One time I was at an airport with other Christian women in Colorado at a leadership conference. I happened to see a US Marine waiting for a flight. He was off in the corner by himself staring at a photo. All of a sudden, I had this overwhelming pull to go over and pray for him. There were people all over, but he was a man, and I was a woman. *What would people think?* After about two-seconds, I lost my worry as conviction hit my personal selfishness. I got out of my seat. I realized this man could be heading into a very harmful situation, one from which he may not return. The very least I could do on his behalf was to offer to pray with him. I motioned to the other five women I was with, and they followed me.

I knelt down on my knees in front of his chair and asked him where he was going and if we could pray for him. He told me he was worried he would never see his seven-year-old daughter again. The rest of the women knelt down too, and we all prayed, right there on the carpet of the airport. Tears in his eyes, he thanked us and then, just like that, they called him to board. If I had waited, or went to the bathroom first to collect my thoughts, I would have missed the opportunity. When the Holy Spirit leads, we need to go!

ARMOR ALERT: Be a Witness

1. **What are you multiplying most in your life?**

2. **Share an experience with your AP/AG about a time you witnessed to someone else. If you have not had the opportunity yet, pray that God would give you many.**

Week 10, Day 4
Discipleship

"Go therefore and make disciples of all the nations, baptizing them in the name of the Father and of the Son and of the Holy Spirit."
—Matthew 28:19

I may have opportunities to witness to others, but that does not mean I see any fruit of my labor. My role in their lives could very well end with a smile, good deed, or a quick conversation about Christ. It could be another's job to disciple that person. God commands us to go and make disciples (Matthew 28:19). If you are a follower of Jesus, you are His disciple. A disciple is one who accepts and assists in spreading the doctrines of another.[12] You have opportunities all around you to disciple others. In fact, you could already be doing it now, and you might not realize to what extent.

The story of Paul and Timothy, in 1 Timothy 1, is a fantastic example of a discipleship relationship. Paul reminds Timothy of his calling and purpose in life and helps him with focus and goals. Paul leads by example of how to fulfill this call (Acts 18:5). Paul is unwavering in his encouragement to press forward in the hard times that are coming. There is no envy or competition between the two because their focus is on the same goal; the genuine interest of seeing others comet o Christ and fulfill their purposes in life.

"Salvation is free, but discipleship costs everything we have."—Billy Graham

We demonstrate we want the best for others when we actually love and care for them. Discipleship happens when we teach, correct, and train others in the love of Christ. Naturally, a Christ-following parent will disciple their children. They will encourage them to spend time with Jesus (an action step) to grow in their personal relationship with Him. Once we love someone, it is hard to reverse it.

The Bible tells us things about heaven, yet He withholds fascinating mysteries. God created heaven, which means He will be there. He is the Light of heaven. It comes from His glory, not the physical sun. If God was, is, and is to come (Revelation 1:8), He will for sure be in heaven with all His people, angels, and awesome creations. We naturally should want to know the Master of heaven deeply if we are going to be in His heavenly house for eternity. He allows us to be a part of His big master plan here on the earth and share in it in heaven after this world passes—what an honor! He gives us a choice to love Him and decide for ourselves if we will accept the blessing of worshiping Him in truth.

Love is a growing choice—and action. Just think if your spouse was forced to love you, and secretly disliked you. I am not talking about the time after a disagreement when we honestly do not like the other person at that moment. I am referring to a constant state of dislike. I do not know any woman that would want to live and spend eternity with forced love. God does not either. He wants our true unwavering love. Just as you would die for your child—the greatest love of all (John 15:13)—so too He requests that depth of our love for Him. Our love for Christ will grow as we spend more time with Him, which will enable us love others more. Jesus loves His people, and when we truly love Him, we will naturally love what He loves. Our hearts will desire to help others because Jesus' love will flow in and through us. This opens the floodgates, the desires, and the opportunities to mentor and disciple others.

ARMOR ALERT: Discipleship Tools Found in the Armor of God

You may or may not be teaching someone else these core values, tools, or spiritual disciplines through the Armor of God right now. Read through the below statements and make notes below each if you are sharing these values, and with who you are sharing them. There are many more ways and areas you can disciple others. Just remember to make Jesus and His Word the center of it all.

- Knowing the truth (Belt of Truth)
- Understanding God's character and becoming like Him (Breastplate of Righteousness)
- Learning how to pray (Shield of Faith)
- Defending and sharing the Gospel (Gospel of Peace)
- Knowing and being empowered by the Holy Spirit (Sword of the Spirit)
- Having assurance of salvation (Helmet of Salvation)

Testimony

"Or do you not know that your body is the temple of the Holy Spirit *who is* in you, whom you have from God, and you are not your own? For you were bought at a price; therefore glorify God in your body and in your spirit, which are God's," (1 Corinthians 6:19-20).

As I read those words at the beginning of this book, it hit me in a way I have never seen it before. I sensed God strongly speaking to my spirit. "I" tried to eat better/lose weight, to feel better about "me" and to gain acceptance and approval from others. However, no matter how hard "I" tried to eat better and move more, "I" could only be so strong for so long. It may take months, weeks or even days, but eventually all the old habits, fears and strongholds that would cause me to make the unhealthy choices would come storming back into my life stronger than ever. My focus was on what I could do. My struggle with weight was not something on which I focused on asking God for help, because after all, it was my poor choices that led me to gain weight.

I felt God strongly impressing on me two things:

1. I am saved by God. I am his temple. I would never desecrate His church, so why am I desecrating the very place He so personally dwells with poor lifestyle choices?
2. My focus for a healthier lifestyle has been off track. It has always been focused on "me" and "my" efforts, on what I feel I will gain once getting to that perfect weight.

I sensed God asking me to hand over all control with my eating habits and lifestyle, to put my focus daily on seeking and obeying Him so that He will get the glory. You know what, He is faithful. I can honestly say that these last several months I have experienced self-control and peace that I know can only come from Him. In my old willpower, I would give in to bad choices daily, sometimes more than once a day. I am experiencing success in weight loss, but even more importantly, He is building my faith on what He can do through me if I am willing to ask!

Kelly Orcutt,
Park View, Iowa

Before You Meet

Take a closer look at your Pre-Evaluation Chart concerning your spiritual health. The condition of your spirit is most important in the grand scheme of life. Take a few minutes and evaluate your week. What did you learn that you put in practice? Be prepared to ask or answer deeper questions with your AP.

Left side of chart: unsure of afterlife, unthankful, unloving, not giving, not witnessing, not professing truth, fake, closed, scared, unholy, not cleaving to God

Right side of chart: saved, peaceful, hopeful, faithful, truthful, righteous, meek, humble, loving, assured, holy, witnessing, forgiving, praying, listening

Trainer Talk

Can you believe you are at the end of another 2-Week Challenge? How is your nutrition and exercise going? How are you going to put on the shield of faith in these weeks ahead? (Look back through the chapters if you can't answer the question yet.)

Remember to look your AP in the eyes and tell her something beautiful about her spiritual health that you admire.

IT'S TIME TO MEET!

SECTION SIX

HELMET OF SALVATION

We have progressed through most of the Armor of God in the past few weeks together, but have a little left to go. The following two weeks puts emphasis on the helmet of salvation and our mental health. We will begin with the 2-Week Mentally Strong Challenge. Read the below verse a few times before continuing. Ask God to help you this week.

"Take the helmet of salvation and the sword of the Spirit,
which is the Word of God" (Ephesians 6:17).

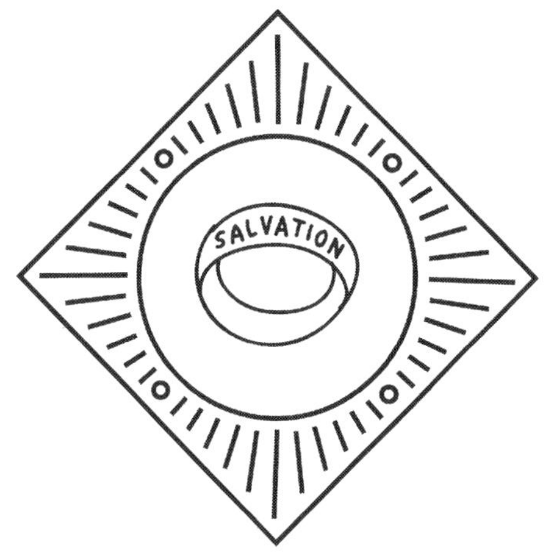

Week 11: Arm Yourself with Salvation
Week 12: Arm Yourself with Mental Health

Health Challenge #5
2-Week Mentally Strong Challenge

This challenge might be harder than all the rest, but I guarantee there will be a bigger reward. Below are spiritual activities to strengthen your mental health:

1. Pray at a different time during the day than normal. Count how many times you can offer up prayers on behalf of others.
2. Randomly stop by at a friend's house that you have not seen for a while; visit, talk or drop off healthy banana bread—even adults like surprises.
3. Specifically, pray for a friend that you are jealous of and ask blessings for them.
4. Visit a friend in the hospital, no matter how uncomfortable it is.
5. Invite a friend out for coffee or dinner.
6. Pray and ask God to bless your enemies.
7. Grab a friend and have a long brisk walk to talk specifically about God.
8. Visit or call an unsaved family member and tell them a Christ-centered testimony.
9. If there is bitterness in your heart towards someone specific, pray for it to leave, but also bless that person with a small gift or card.
10. Try to take a fitness class that you have never tried before, meet someone new, and bring God into the conversation somehow by the end of class.
11. Stop off at a bookstore and pick up a Christ-centered book someone suggested (then make daily time to read it).
12. Write a letter (snail mail style) to an older or aged friend.
13. Ask your church where you can help in an unusual way (ask others to join you).
14. Call a close friend just to tell them you love and cherish them.
15. Pick a character out of the Bible and study him or her (then apply it to your life).
16. Cook something you have never tried before, and eat it with family and friends.
17. Create something—cookbook, journal, address book, floral arrangement, scarf, picture collage—and then give it away to someone undeserving.
18. Volunteer to serve; at a local food pantry, a widow in church, with neighborhood weeding, at the Red Cross, at a homeless shelter, at a local school—even if you don't have kids, with Big Brothers Big Sisters, as a Lunch Buddy to a kid without a mom or dad, at a library, at a retirement home, or by watching kids for a local Bible study, etc.
19. Join a Christ-centered group, online blog, social media group, library book club, fitness class, scrapbook club, older adult center, or Bible study (like Community Bible Study or Bible Study Fellowship, or one in your church).
20. Start a Bible-focused group (an area MOPS, Bible study, or a Christ-centered book club) in your neighborhood.

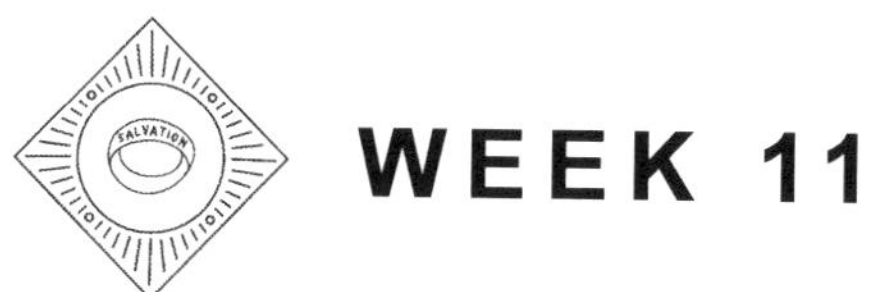

WEEK 11

ARM YOURSELF WITH SALVATION

Week 11, Day 1
Helmet of Salvation

"And take the helmet of salvation, and the sword of the Spirit, which is the Word of God."
—Ephesians 6:17

A helmet protects our heads just as salvation protects our minds. Knowing what we believe will help us make better decisions, stand our ground when things are bad, and encourage others. God tells us to stay rooted, daily renewing our minds with the Scriptures. The Bible is not like an elementary school spelling test where we can memorize the information the night before and forget after the test. We shouldn't read a few verses one time and be done with it. Reading the Bible is a lifestyle and gives us a daily roadmap to follow. Even though we will never know, this side of heaven, all aspects of the cross (because it is unfathomable that our God would send His Son to this earth to be tortured and die), we do know God loves us so very much. He blessed us with the ability to be free agents, either longing to spend our life with Him or deciding we can do things on our own without Him.

Just like our faith is placed simply in the rising and setting of the sun, we need simple faith in Jesus as our Savior to save us from eternity without Him. This love is not logical at times, especially when we encounter the roadblocks of doubt placed by the enemy, like if God loved us, why do bad things happen? Our problems are not because of God, but because of the absence of Him. If you ever have a crisis of faith, questioning whether all of Christ's promises are true, ask yourself if the enemy was allowed in through a possible crack in your heart.

"Our problems aren't because of God, but because of the absence of Him."

Knees shaking, while standing in battle, not knowing if death will consume you that very hour is beyond terrifying. Believers know where they are going when death claims their natural bodies. They know they do not have anything to lose on this earth compared to joy everlasting in heaven with the Creator of all. Some acquaintances have told me when I mention Jesus it rubs them the wrong way, and even makes them angry and agitated. Some have said they feel guilty inside or their hearts start racing at the mention of Jesus' name (I love these honest folks! I then know exactly how to pray for them).

There is a clear explanation why people have internal reactions to the name of Jesus. He is the real deal. This war with spiritual forces makes hearts and spirits respond in some way or another. Jesus is the standard and supreme universal authority. He is the way, the truth, and the life. When anyone speaks this ultimate Truth, the opposite side shudders. "It is a fearful thing to fall into the hands of the living God" (Hebrews 10:31, KJV). God created our spirits, so when we are going against Him, something inside is unsettled. Likewise, when the Holy Spirit pulls us to Him, something in our spirits is intrigued, afraid, nervous, or even convicted.

Luke 10:19 shows that we have the power and authority to overcome all the powers of the enemy, and nothing will harm us. Nothing will hurt us eternally, not even Satan himself. We can resist the enemy, and he will flee from us because there is power and authority in the name of Jesus (James 4:7). It is the most powerful Name in all of history and in the spiritual world, which is why there is so much opposition to it. In the name of Jesus, demons flee. No other person's name can do this. No other name has more power than Jesus' does. Not only did Jesus alter the entire history of the world, the very mention of His Name still alters human spirits and sends demons fleeing. The reason brave souls are not scared of death is that they have their helmet of salvation on securely. They know deep down the demons of this holy war cannot touch them. Their spirit is completely secure from the enemy and eternal death.

We all need saving from our sin because we all fall short of God. No one is perfect, but those who do not think they sin or need saving from their sins will not see the value in salvation. Salvation is our crown, our helmet. When we find the truth, no one can take that away from us. It protects us from lies and fiery darts from the enemy. Just knowing Scripture will not secure salvation alone. Believing, trusting, and having faith in Jesus does.

Have you ever been so stressed you sweat blood? I thought I was when giving natural birth to twins, but even that was not anything close to what others have been through, especially Jesus. Before the crucifixion, as Jesus prayed in the Garden of Gethsemane, the disciple and physician Luke noted, "And being in anguish, He prayed more earnestly, and his sweat was like drops of blood falling to the ground" (Luke 22:44). Luke, a physician and well-educated man, seems to have made careful observation by profession. Although this medical condition is relatively rare, there have been actual cases of it. The clinical term is hematohidrosis. Around the sweat glands, there are multiple blood vessels in a net-like form. Under the pressure of immense stress, the vessels constrict. Then, as the anxiety passes, the blood vessels dilate to the point of rupture. The blood goes into the sweat glands. As the sweat glands are producing a lot of sweat, it pushes the blood to the surface, coming out as droplets of blood mixed with sweat.[13]

Jesus was going to experience immense physical pain. Being the Son of God, He knew what He was physically facing—one of the most horrible forms of capital punishment ever. His body was also fully human, and He would feel everything as intensely as we humans could. However, it is doubtful this was the source of his severe stress. Jesus knew the suffering would be momentary. Besides, others have faced this similar physical fate of torture and the cross. I believe the vast weight upon Jesus was the knowledge that He would soon bear the terrible burden of taking the guilt of sin for all upon Himself—your sins and mine.

Sin separates us from God, and although Jesus never sinned, when He took the burden of our horrible sins, the Father turned His face. Jesus said, "Father, why have you forsaken Me?" I believe this is the source of the anxiety and drops of blood coming from His pores. Jesus died and was separated from the Father so that we would not have to go through that. If Jesus sweated blood in the face of separation from the Father for three days, that should tell us something dangerously terrifying about dying without God forever. It was a spiritual sacrifice, a spiritual sacrifice we will never completely wrap our minds around on this earth. He came back to life to show us all He is God and has the final victory forever.

"If we say that we have no sin, we deceive ourselves, and the truth is not in us. If we confess our sins, He is faithful and just to forgive us our sins and to cleanse us from all unrighteousness. If we say that we have not sinned, we make Him a liar, and His Word is not in us" (1 John 1:8-10).

ARMOR ALERT: Your Journey to Jesus

Many people helped shape and disciple me into the woman I am today. We can all pinpoint special moments that had the most impact on us. These encouraging nuggets along our journey in life are a testimony to the faithful work of Jesus. I believe these little testimonies are not to be secrets.

1. **Share one personal memory within your salvation testimony.**

2. **I am challenging you this week to share pieces, or all, of your testimony with your AP/AG or someone else that has never heard it before. If you have never written it out before, write it this week.**

Week 11, Day 2
Organization of the Soul

"And do not be conformed to this world, but be transformed by the renewing of your mind, that you may prove what is that good and acceptable and perfect will of God."
—Romans 12:2

If we own our home, we take necessary steps in that ownership as we commit to the purchase, perform any maintenance, and fill it with things we love. We take care of it. We protect it at all costs. We take more pride and time with our investment versus if we just rented space from someone else, like an apartment. When we own our belief and desires, we will take more pride and make any needed investments in it. We cannot rent our salvation, looking for the next space to house our hearts. We need to take our time and know why we believe what we believe, and never put our beliefs up for rent.

I invest in my soul in many ways, just like in your 2-Week Challenge with spiritual disciplines. Personally, I connect with God through prayer, meditation, and reading His Word most. I feel this is how to take care of my faith, own it, repair it, groom it, and grow in it. I have heard others are close to God and fulfill the desires of their souls by being in nature or dancing. God carefully creates His people with different passions (*amen to that—can you imagine everyone loving chips and salsa? We'd run out!)*. When I connect with God in the morning, I focus more on my daily living, dreams, ambitions, and goals, than when I wait until the end of the day. This enables and helps me to grow into the woman I am striving to be, because God knows, I am not that complete woman yet.

Scripture gives me so much instruction on a daily basis of what I need to be doing and how, no matter what my personal goals are. It is fascinating how it applies so much. I can crack open the Bible and it is as if God wrote those very words for me at that moment to read (I've grasped the reason why it's called the Living Word). I know beyond any doubt when I limit my daily Bible reading for even a few days, something happens inside and gives me ill feelings, I act more like a child and demand my agenda. The Bible keeps me on the straight and narrow in more than just daily living but in my very soul.

"We cannot rent our salvation, looking for the next space to house our hearts. We need to take our time and know why we believe what we believe, and never put our beliefs up for rent."

God did not leave us here blind on the earth with no daily plan of action. He gave us practical steps to follow for our soul care by obeying His directives. If you want to take the first step in knowing His will for you, follow His commands. Romans 12:2 says, "Do not conform to the pattern of this world, but be transformed by the renewing of your mind. Then you will be able to test and approve what God's will is—His good, pleasing and perfect will." If I focused on what other people thought of me that day in the airport in

Colorado, I would have gone to the restroom to collect my thoughts first and would have missed the opportunity to pray over a soldier. I believe it was God's plan that I was there during those very minutes.

I want to record on every page of this book how important it is to meet up with God daily. It brings peace to my soul, my perspective changes, and my heart softens. It helps me understand the bigger picture and the simple reason God would save a wretch like me. When I spend quality time with Him, I feel an inner connection that is unexplainable. We can't sustain a constant search for the new idea, or thing, to help fill our soul with contentment. Spending time with God and reading His Word is the way to do this correctly. Do no skip out on the most important meeting of the day—time with Him.

ARMOR ALERT: Get Organized

Below are several directives from Scripture, and all are moral codes written in each of our hearts to engage. They are not just suggestions to make us feel warm and fuzzy inside, although they do. These action steps help in the spiritual and physical worlds, and they will contribute to our health and bring strength to our bones. They will shape us into who we want to be—women after God's own heart.

Look up at least two Scripture references from a topic below in which you feel you could be more organized, and then make a goal to be active about what you read.

1. **Are you productive?** He tells us to work hard at all we do and do it unto the Lord, not to please others: Colossians 3:23; Genesis 2:15; Proverbs 16:3; 2 Timothy 3:16-17; Philippians 4:13.
    a. When we do not work, we become lazy and are unproductive, and then people cannot trust us to get things done on time.
    b. Are you living to please God or man more?

2. **Are you resting with God?** Jesus demonstrates Himself to have rest and moments of meditation and quiet times alone with the Father: Joshua 1:8; Psalm 1:1-6, 46:10; Philippians 4:8; Matthew 6:6.
    a. When we do not have moments of meditation or rest, we stress, overwork, and may snap at others.
    b. When was the last time you sat and prayed longer than 10-minutes without your mind making to-do lists?

3. **Are you moral?** He directs us to flee from evil: 1 Thessalonians 5:22; Ephesians 5:11; 1 Peter 5:8; James 1:14.
    a. We get in trouble spiritually and physically when we hang out in bad places.
    b. Are you morally defined by social surroundings or God's?

4. **Are you social?** He desires us to have interaction with others socially, like going to church: Hebrews 10:25; John 13:34; Romans 12:5; Colossians 3:16.
    a. When we do not connect with others, we may deviate from accountability, be depressed, lonely, or off the right spiritual path.
    b. Do you interact with those outside your social and economic circle?

5. **Are you making disciples?** He tells us to train up others, and encourage and lead them towards Christ through mentoring: Matthew 28:19; 2 Timothy 2:2; Mark 3:14; Luke 10:1-3; James 5:16; Hebrews 10:25.
    a. When we do not invest in others, we focus more on ourselves, the "I."
    b. When was the last time you mentored, discipled, or led someone to Christ?

Week 11, Day 3
Immortal Entitlement

"What causes quarrels and what causes fights among you? Is it not this, that your passions are at war within you?"
—James 4:1, ESV

When I am late for something important, impatience grows up from my belly right through the top of my head. My mind starts telling me I am more important than the other parents dropping off their kids at school, and thus I should have the right of way. *Why is my mind commanding my personal relevance above all others? Does that classify me as impatient and prideful?* Entitlement issues rob us of patience, peace, joy, and love for others. It is growing right alongside our waistline and destroying our health. We know our mental state ties to our emotions just as much as our physical body entertains pleasures. If someone is hurting and hemorrhaging, before long, more health areas bleed and suffer as well.

Angry marital fights break out when we feel we are so right and our spouse is so dead wrong. Arms crossed, heels dug deep, we will not move from our belief in the situation. Again, this proves that the "I" is alive and well and is ready to wage war. We have a hard time remembering we can agree to disagree without the snap, snarl, and squawk. Tabling the conversation until things simmer down, so the boiling pot does not tip and burn someone we love, is sometimes easier said than done. When we feel the "I" is not considered highly by our loved ones, or our personal desires and preferences are not met, we tend to find a resolution the "I" way. Some break relationship commitments when needs are not met, which leads to crushing consequences.

Our minds can create entitlement problems with just one little negative thought. We have all seen it demonstrated many a time—a guy is in a hurry and expects faster service at the store check out line. He does not receive it in his timeline, so he causes a ruckus. All others watching are in the same boat—they too are inconvenienced—but for some reason, this guy believes he is entitled to have priority over others. This scene happens more and more in our society as the time ticks on. Our incredibly blessed lifestyles are lending so many comforts that we cannot seem to handle any little discomfort. We pretty much have our needs met in this modern world with temperature-controlled shelter, fine clothing, more than enough food, and even more than enough clean drinking water, not to mention all the other trinkets that consume us.

Of course, we might not think we have the comforts so deserved and entitled. After all, someone will always have greener grass on their side of the fence—and the cycle of entitlement continues. Our self-deserved thought process about what we want, when we want it, and how we want it rings louder with every new appliance and technology breakthrough When we are afforded these privileges repetitively, it is hard to imagine living without them. If our electricity has momentarily halted, it can cause some to hyperventilate. They cannot seem to function for those four hours in the storm without power (and that's because I have walked in these shoes!).

I think back periodically to that dreadful day, September 11th, 2001, and the stories we heard following. Some spilled coffee on their pants on the way to work and turned around to change, thus missing the entire tragedy. A lady's alarm did not go off, and she was running late to work, so late that she did not make it there before things went tragic. A dad had to stay home from work with his sick child because the mom was out of town. God has a plan for our lives, and when things go wrong, we need to stop and realize there just might be another reason behind the so-called inconvenience. If our food is not coming fast enough or we are catching every red light on the morning commute, God might be at work behind the scenes. If the purpose is learning patience, or not ending up sandwiched in a massive pile up on the road, we must learn to trust, obey, and enjoy every second of every moment—wherever God holds us up.

Kids think they have a lot of time left before their earthly body expires. They feel immortal because they have their whole lives to live. *I still think the same way as an adult.* The grave sounds so far away, and because of it, we can easily postpone things to a later time. We could push back getting a mammogram, mending a friendship, spending time with our kids, eating healthier, or investing in our future financially. Tomorrow is unknown, and we expect the sun to rise just like all the days before. There will be a time when we realize we pushed things off too long. Regardless if we lived a life of reckless living or proactive measures, we will all one day meet our Creator. Our goal right now, at this very hour, is to be as ready as we can spiritually to meet Him. If you left this earth in a blink of an eye today, would you be at peace to meet God?

ARMOR ALERT: Hang up on Entitlements

As you wait and stand in long lines at the store, do you tap your foot, cross your arms, complain, or grumble in your mind? If so, this could be a good exercise to experiment and pray over.

1. **Ask God to show you how to think less of your personal importance and place it on someone else. Use the suggestions below as examples.**
   a. Allow someone else to go before you in line.
   b. Ask God for opportunities to drive with less road rage.
   c. Think more highly of someone else and pray for them.
   d. Ask God to protect your mind from getting caught in a jealousy battle.
   e. Pray you would not seek out your personal gain in a situation.

2. **Share specific conquering moments with your AP/AG next time you meet.**

Trainer Talk
Do you think you have any entitlement issues? I have had plenty. I'm asking God to continue helping me focus on Him instead of myself (this is a hard one to be good at). We all struggle with mental garbage at times, the goal is to give it to God and struggle less with each passing hour. You may now be more comfortable sharing your faith with a deeper understanding of salvation. Trust and rest in God's pure love for you. This should make your mind be at peace and your heart smile.

Week 11, Day 4
Time Investments

"A joyful heart is good medicine, but a crushed spirit dries up the bones."
—Proverbs 17:22, ESV

Over-commitment is stressful and leads to worry, which leads to a depressed, overloaded, aged, and an emotional hot mess of a woman. These feelings control our physical actions and can make us waste our week of exercise on an entire tub of ice cream. When we enter the day on our own strength with a paper sword in one hand and a cup of coffee in the other, we will not be as equipped as God wants us to be. Putting God first in our day will help us in these battles from the enemy.

Can you recognize when you are stressed? Some of us can't tell when stress is slapping us in the face. There are patterns I now recognize when I stress—I do not look at my kids or husband in the eyes and am short with my tongue. I also notice my volume level goes up about two notches and I get agitated easily. When this starts to happen, I start waving my big red flag of stress, which can come on quick and at the most inopportune times. Stress eats away at our minds, controls our emotions and starts to take over our actions. It is a vicious cycle that needs recognizing and treatment.

One area that brings on stress for me is unresolved conflict. I think about the issue over and over in my mind, and soon all my energy is lost to it. It can even be minimal in the grand scheme of things, but my mind begins to paint a much larger painting on an invisible canvas. My kids ask a simple question as my mind is preoccupied and I reply with a lapse in judgment. *I'm sure I could get an "amen" from someone reading this.* It is no secret stress attacks us in many different avenues.

Stress doesn't saturate our minds when we focus on Christ. When I have unresolved conflict, I should immediately pray and ask God to give me clarity of thought, a sound mind, a solution, perfect timing, and a good attitude. It is as if my lapse in judgment is finding me out in all sorts of areas. The "I" gets the best of me and almost withholds me from praying about it. When I have reached this stage, I realize my soul is unorganized, my priorities are messy, and my time with God is lacking.

Investing time in the Lord is truly the best time spent and the best thing to consume our minds. Sometimes it is hard to be still and just take time for Him, but remember that He rests and renews our minds and brings us refreshment in our soul. I do honestly feel like He multiplies my time when I start my day with Him. I seem to get more done in less time, with more joy, as He blesses me because I sought Him first.

"Too much to do and not enough time to do it!" rolls off the lips of many frequently. There is an easy answer to this predicament. "Be still, and know that I am God; I will be exalted among the nations, I will be exalted in the earth" (Psalm 46:10). Make time for God first, then yourself. It is as easy as that. Just be still. Some call this quiet time, devotion, or meditation. When we are still and wait on God to show us, tell us or prompt something within our hearts, there is renewing within our spirits. We are allowing connection with Him. For some, being still means yoga, sleeping, watching TV or reading a book, but what about just being still and doing nothing except waiting on God in the quiet of your mind in your special place? For me, my physical body wants to be constantly moving. It is very hard for me to just sit still.

Since I was young, I would rise before everyone else in my home. I would not even need an alarm clock. I would keep myself busy doing everything and anything. I have been this way my entire life. I have never required a lot of sleep, although that requirement is changing a bit these past few years. However, I was very convicted when I read the words in the Scripture, "Be still," because that was so not me. I never realized I was experiencing any form of stress from never resting until I clung to that verse. I sat and, doing nothing physically, cleared my mind of my situations in life and asked God to fill it with His plans and thoughts for me. Never can I recall a time I felt so refreshed. I was simply stress-free.

I realized I had to train myself to be still, as unnatural as that sounds. I had to stop consuming my mind with things of this world. Instead of snuggling up on the couch with technology, I had to train myself to snuggle up with God and His Word. At first, I felt like I had to hurry through this time because I had so much to do elsewhere. This was selfishness on my part. I prayed for anxiety to leave so I could spend whatever time was needed on my relationship with Him. The specific thing I asked God for was to multiply my time and give me clarity of thought.

God has granted my requests more times than I can count. I frequently am asked by others how I do all that I do. Simply put, God multiplies my time if I give Him the first fruits of my day. When I feel stress, anxiety, or a lack of having it together, I ask Him to organize my day, and help me take things off my plate that I don't need.

ARMOR ALERT: Prioritization

1. **Make a list of your *outside-the-home* monthly obligations/duties.** (Carpools, committees, jobs, church volunteering, coaching, etc.)

2. **Now add your required *in-home* monthly duties and possibly list the different hats you wear.** (Housework, yard work, caregiver, wife, mom, roommate, sibling, etc.)

3. **Look at the two lists above. Is there anything you think God is calling you to step away from or prioritize better in your life that is creating stress?** (Pray about this and share your solution with your AP/AG.)

Trainer Talk

Mental challenges can play tricks on us, like making us think we are not doing as good of a job as we could, or making us question why we devote all this hard work when we are not seeing results. Our minds are super powerful (but not as powerful as God). Be encouraged that you can power through your times of mental battles with God. He is your strength so don't feel like you have to fight all by yourself.

Before You Meet
Take the Helmet of Salvation

Moment for Meditation

Lord Almighty,

You are more than enough for me. You are holy, wonderful, and powerful. Thank you for the plan of salvation. Help me never take for granted what You accomplished at the cross. Help me never forget how salvation is priceless. Today, I need your strength and help to be even more amazing at what you are calling me to do.

I put on the belt of truth. I ask You to put truth on my lips and in my heart at all times. I ask that You put the truth of the Gospel around me and never let me forget it.

I put on the breastplate of righteousness and ask you to guard my heart against any enemy darts that may come my way. Protect my emotions and guard my mouth.

I put on the Gospel of peace. Guide my steps today so I may be a blessing and share boldly through my words and actions.

I take up the shield of faith and ask for strength and courage. Build my faith so I can do everything You call me to do with complete excellence.

I take the helmet of salvation and ask You to guard my mind against garbage from the enemy. Help me to recognize attacks and to be prepared to combat them when they come. Thank you for your armor and unconditional love. In the name of Jesus, amen.

IT'S TIME TO MEET!

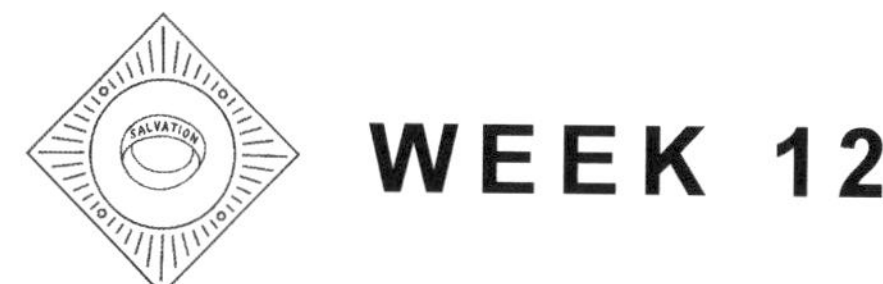

WEEK 12

ARM YOURSELF WITH MENTAL HEALTH

Week 12, Day 1
Character Counts

"Therefore, as the elect of God, holy and beloved, put on tender mercies, kindness, humility, meekness, longsuffering; bearing with one another, and forgiving one another, if anyone has a complaint against another; even as Christ forgave you, so you also must do."
—Colossians 3:12-13

Some of you may have one child who is a little more trustworthy than their sibling. One of my twins normally forgets to bring important notes home from school, but all of my other kids can easily handle this. I could leave that same twin at home with full trust before I could leave some of the other siblings. One child never abuses their phone privileges while other siblings happen to get them taken away frequently. The different levels of trust are reflections of their characters.

Our various character traits are one of the most precious blessings God has ever given us. Character is the way someone thinks, feels, and behaves—someone's personality.[14] It defines who we are to others and ourselves. It shows up in moments of trial when wounded, and present when nothing else is left. Character is hard to build and easy to lose. We all face daily opportunities to improve or weaken our character. God wants to mold us into an even more tremendous woman of God.

"Character is like a tree and reputation like a shadow. The shadow is what we think of it; the tree is the real thing."—Abraham Lincoln

We can manufacture the fruit of the Spirit in our lives for only so long (love, joy, peace, patience, etc), because the Bible says we need the Spirit to achieve this. Some can manipulate others, such as being nice to their kids in public and treat them poorly at home. God knows the condition of our heart and true character. He knows when we manipulate, cheat, steal, or have ill thoughts. If we recognize signs of our character producing rotten fruit, this is our opportunity to repent and seek after Him for a solution.

We have that person in our lives we would like imitate in character. They may be able to have peace in the midst of a trail or never share a juicy detail about someone else. The character of God is what we should strive to imitate. Paul writes of the Armor of God with the breastplate second as a needed piece in this spiritual war. It protects our hearts—our emotional health. Without a physically protected heart, we would die. Likewise, without righteousness, we would die spiritually.

You can take this entire week to work on allowing the Holy Spirit to come in and mend or impart anything you need. This week your focus is: to sharpen your character through the Holy Spirit and not on your own. He wants to bless and mold you into even a more beautiful warrior inside and out. I encourage you to take times out this week and just rest and listen, to the Holy Spirit. If you're not sure if He is communicating something to you, read the Bible. John 14:26 is clear that the Comforter (Counselor, Helper, Intercessor, Advocate), the Holy Spirit, will cause you to recall (will bring to your remembrance) everything Jesus has told you. The Bible is the living Word of God, and it speaks to our spirit's when we read it and ask the Holy Spirit for counsel. Pray and ask Him to speak to you and that you would recognize things when revealed.

Obeying and listening to God builds our character and faith.

ARMOR ALERT: Character Cleanse

Take some time to think about your personal character, and please do not rush through it. Think about traits with which you are super proud, ones with which you are okay, and others that may need improvement. Dig deep and think about how you treat others and how they respond to you.

1. **List the character traits you are strong in.**

2. **What character traits do you desire to be wonderful in?**

3. **What one action step could you take to start improving the character traits you listed in answer to number 2?**

Active	Energetic	Pleasing
Adventurous	Enthusiastic	Polite
Affectionate	Forgiving	Popular
Aggressive	Hard-working	Positive
Ambitious	Healthy	Punctual
Committed	Helpful	Righteous
Communicative	Honest	Silly
Compassionate	Leader	Sincere
Confident	Lively	Sly
Consistent	logical	Smart
Courageous	Loving	Truthful
Easygoing	Playful	Unselfish
Eloquent	Pleasant	Wise
Encouraging		

Week 12, Day 2
Conquering Mental Assaults

"...whose minds the god of this age has blinded, who do not believe, lest the light of the gospel of the glory of Christ, who is the image of God, should shine on them."
—2 Corinthians 4:4

Mental battles have plagued us from the beginning of time. There are countless Bible verses and proverbs, chants, and the like that revolve around positive and proactive thinking. Humans need life direction, wisdom to follow, and something to cling to that will lend guidance and help in troubled areas. After all, we all have a story and every story has a plot. These plots have a lot to do with relationships. Friendship fallouts can plague our minds with internal warring that block us from spiritual communication.

Internal wars have many names—stress, anxiety, depression, comparison, compulsion, jealousy, and fatigue to name a few. At times, this battlefield in our minds can bring us to our knees. The struggle of not taking that extra slice of cheesecake, not being jealous of a neighbor's new car upgrade, not engaging in revenge when a co-worker passes you up the ladder, or not being depressed for no apparent reason can cause unnecessary garbage. We can't afford to be held in bondage to this cycle of mental war, along with its joy-zapping struggles. God has a plan to free us from our internal warring and pain.

When we allow negativity to churn and replay in our minds, it slowly allows a foothold for the enemy. Our guard is down, so negativity can slither in and settle down. Once it gets cozy, it plants deep roots. Why do we sometimes find ourselves secretively, and compulsively, shoveling that last handful of junk food in our mouths? The enemy whispers lies that we need it, yearn for it, and have to have it now. We feel hopeless to resist the beckoning to come back to the feeding trough, even though we are not hungry and know we should not eat it. This spiritual and mental communication is taking place and is controlling. It is propelling us to do things we do not even want to do.

There is a lot more behind trying to resist Satan and his demons than mere willpower. Some battles cannot be turned on and off with the flip of a switch. They assault us regardless of how hard we try to stop them. Even the strongest-willed leaders cannot conquer some mental battles all by themselves. We need Christ so desperately. His Word renews our minds and helps place things in perspective. He helps stop the rewind, the negative mental garbage. It is the Lord's power that does the fixing, the healing, and the regeneration (John 14:27), not tools from this world, like yoga meditation. We are called to put on the helmet of salvation, not just relaxing music to calm our nerves.

Our physical bodies can respond in different ways when stressed. Some lose hair and others find more gray ones. Some sleep and others go without seeing their bedroom for days. Stress can cause many issues deeper than physical ailments. We read earlier how one health derailment leads to another. When we head into stressful times, we can allow anything, such as food, television, anger, or sleep, to be our antidotes. We can combat these failing remedies internally if we prepare ourselves with some pre-stress tools found in the Armor of God.

You have learned to allow God's truths to ring in your heart and that you do not need food to comfort you (nutritional health). Ask God for righteousness to prevail in your life at all costs, even if you feel like you will lose out (emotional health). Read God's Word and renew your mind daily to build faith in your heart and increase your confidence in His love for you (spiritual and mental health). Combat negativity with peaceful responses and ask Him for protection over your relationships, because fallouts with friends can lead to huge stressors (social health). Constantly ask God to be the center of your life, even if that means saying it out loud to Him in prayer.

Maybe you are not in any mental washing cycle right now, but eventually, our minds question and counteract some of what our hearts desire. This is why we should renew our minds daily with Christ. Some will try to renew their minds in other ways. Take the popular Indian tradition, Yoga. Yoga is more than physical exercise; it has a meditative and spiritual core.[15] One of the six major orthodox schools of Hinduism, or Yoga, which has its own epistemology and metaphysics, is closely related to Hindu Samkhya philosophy.[16] People do yoga to practice and fight hard to relax and control their mind as they connect with spiritual oneness and their bodies. The practices of meditation and body awareness are not the problem; it is with whom they are channeling their oneness.

God explicitly tells us to meditate on Him, and not on our bodies or anyone other than Him. We can have body awareness and control it, stretch it, exercise it, make it move, and sleep; however, the importance of any activity is where our heart is while we are performing it. Are we out to only please others or please God? God's Word says in all we do, do it to the glory of God (1 Corinthians 10:31). Some do not like to use the word "yoga" because of its origin. Use the words "deep stretching" instead.

We cannot entertain allowing the actions of our minds even being allowed to open to unknown spiritual forces as we connect in oneness with the universe in a calming fitness class, chanting to an energy force that is not of God. Our spiritual connections should only be with God. He makes this clear in His Word (Exodus 20:3; Deuteronomy 4:24, 5:7). A successful exercise regimen is to perform deep stretching exercises while you place your thoughts and focus on Him. "In all your ways acknowledge Him, and He shall direct your paths" (Proverbs 3:6).

Our minds are one tricky, misunderstood, and brilliant component of our beings. We do not know all the complexities of how the different spiritual forces communicate with us, or how some have access, and some do not. We need the helmet of salvation to protect us in battle from mental assaults. If He says we need this helmet, we should use it. One of my favorite Scriptures I arm myself with is Hebrews 4:12-13, "For the Word of God is living and powerful, and sharper than any two-edged sword, piercing even to the division of soul and spirit, and of joints and marrow, and is a discerner of the thoughts and intents of the heart. And there is no creature hidden from His sight…" (NKJV).

ARMOR ALERT: Connect with God

1. **Today, take time to connect with God and specifically ask Him to show you if you are connecting with something else besides Him.**

2. **Please talk to your AP/AG about any mental assaults you might be allowing to take place—known or unknown.** (There may be differences of opinions, so please always refer to the Word of God as your source to follow.)

Week 12, Day 3
Serving up Some Stew

"...above all, taking the shield of faith with which you will be able to quench all the fiery darts of the wicked one. And take the helmet of salvation."
—Ephesians 6:16-17

I often wondered why people use the word "stew" when they are mad at someone else until I made some homemade stew myself. I was upset, so I got out my pot and threw in my emotions. I let it simmer for a long while, but it appeared there were not enough ingredients in it, as it began to burn. So after some more thinking, I added additional ingredients—anger, sadness, depression, and ill thoughts. Now I was cooking. I had successfully made my very own stew. I got bored watching it, so I left for a while. Then something jogged my memory, and I realized my stew was still simmering. I came back, and it was just like I left it, but I needed to add more ingredients, like bitterness, imaginations, and unforgiveness, so it would not burn again. The more we think about things over and over with no solution, the larger the stew becomes in the end. If left on high, the stew will boil over and burn any bystanders.

Mind replay. When a relationship hits a speed bump, and a breakdown occurs, I am one to keep the mental tape replaying over and over until I can drum up enough sense of why things went south. When my rewinds aren't focused on solutions, it leads to despondent thoughts, stressed living, and a lack of self-confidence, to name a few. These unhealthy rewind mind games are a ploy from the enemy, who can destroy friendships and zap joy. Arm yourself with the helmet of salvation and stop the damaging mind replays.

There are times when a replay of a disagreement needs to happen, such as finding a solution to a problem. It allows us to reassess the situation. Sometimes, as I replay a conversation, I realize it was received out of context. This gives me the opportunity to correct things by going back to the person with better clarity of thought. I have learned firsthand that sometimes we have a short window to make amends before the hourglass runs out. Once the time is gone, it is much harder to fix a hairy situation.

We cannot ignore someone's feelings, no matter how right we feel we are. Sometimes the problem is an intentional disagreement and other times it is an entirely unintentional disaster. When we realize we hurt someone's feelings, we should rush to apologize, rejecting the "I," by bringing humility of heart and kicking pride to the curb. We can pretend nothing happened, justify actions, and never reconcile, hoping time will heal things by itself, but God does not call us to ignore others (Colossians 3:12-14). He tells us to forgive, be tenderhearted, and compassionate.

Pride can stand in the way of correcting relationship fallouts. Of course, we won't always notice pride blockading healthy relationships, but onlookers sure see it. Pride is a paper shield made from our very own handiwork plastered across our chest—and we parade around with it like peacocks. We can freely ask God to reveal pride in our life. When it's exposed, our job is to repent of it and ask Him to help us notice if it sneaks back in.

We can have confidence that He will help us have less mental rewinds. We need to stand firm in our belief of the Scriptures. Take the shield of faith and say with your mouth, and believe in your heart, what the Bible says is truth. Repeat His promises and renew your mind with them. Ask the Holy Spirit to fill you and lead you. Ask God for more faith, belief, and wisdom. The Bible promises God will give it to us if we ask (James 1:5).

ARMOR ALERT: Internal Warring

1. **Answer these questions in your heart.**
    a. Are you engaged in depressing rewinds from past hurts?
    b. How can knowing God's salvation help you not make stew?
    c. Does your mind have control over your actions?

2. **If you are ready to share a possible situation that is constantly on replay, then be prepared and open up with your AP/AG. Pray together over the situation and ask for a solution.**

Trainer Talk
I have faith you are excelling at your challenges. Are you checking in on your AP with her challenges? Are you working hard, or hardly working on your physical goals? We have a few weeks left together and I can't wait for you to dig into these next chapters. Devote your discipline to finish this program with excellence. Don't throw in the towel on any challenge. Start handing out more towels to your AP and encourage her to continue with excellence too.

Week 12, Day 4
Performance Treadmill

"But each one is tempted when he is drawn away by his own desires and enticed."
—James 1:14

On the last day of creation, God said, "Let Us make man in Our image, in Our likeness," (Genesis 1:26). He finished His work with a personal touch. We are unique among all God's handiwork, fearfully and beautifully made, having both a material body and an immaterial soul/spirit. This likeness is a specialty of our human creation and sets us apart from the animal world, fits us for the dominion God intended us to have over the earth (Genesis 1:28), and enables us to commune with our Maker differently than anything else. Created as rational agents, we can reason and choose. We are a reflection of God's intellect and freedom. Anytime we read or write a book, paint a landscape, play in a symphony, decide to exercise, or pray and communicate with our Maker—animals cannot do all of this. God saw all He had made and called it, "very good" (Genesis 1:31).

When Eve took the fruit of the forbidden tree and gave to Adam, sin entered the world. Think about this for a moment. What did Eve take? Fruit! The first sin ever committed is linked with food. This forbidden fruit was symbolic of everything sin would include. Is it possible to say food sins have been attached to us ever since the Fall of humanity? Food was the very thing God hung on the cursed tree, and the enemy knows it as well.

Eve was intrigued and lured in first with the exceptionally beautiful fruit. It could have been shiny and luscious—one way to get a woman's attention. Food was a downfall in the garden, and it is still one today. Most women are attracted when there is bling, shiny sequins, or beautiful chocolate truffles on display. Our sinful nature gets excited and urges us to desire things that we cannot have. I believe this is why God commands us not to covet things—listed in the Ten Commandments.

That must have been some battle going on inside Eve's mind as she contemplated listening to the crooked serpent or keeping trust in God. Eve mentally processed what was presented, then decided and engaged by taking it off the tree. She physically placed it to her lips and ate, then also shared it with Adam. One thing led to the next. She could have only thought about it and chosen not to engage, but she did not. By merely thinking on it, the engagement became that much easier to act on. We can apply this to anything in our personal lives.

Sometimes sin can lure women and men in very differently. Adam might have passed up on a shiny fruit, but maybe not an 'off limits' wild rhinoceros he would have loved to ride. The differing intrigue points are one area where our weaknesses shine brightest. Sometimes when our weaknesses are on display, we scurry to hide them—and think we do a good job of covering them up (just like the naked couple in the garden). We can do a good job covering up insecurities with external coverings (does wallpaper ring a bell?).

Colossians 3:2 tells us to set our minds and think on things above, things pertaining to God. Society has us trained that to be considered beautiful or healthy, our upper thighs should not be touching, and our chests should stick out farther than our rear ends. Our fellow humans distort God's "made in His perfect image" view as they redefine what God deems beautiful. God made you very good, which in my definition means beautiful, amazing, wonderful, and breathtaking! You might not feel like it all the time, but remember *who* made you, and the likeness in which you were created. Think about the way your body is knit together, cell by cell, the way your blood flows in and out as your heart pumps, and the way your body moves or how it digests food. God created you with pure Awesomeness! There is thoughtful design in the most logical way. No matter if a freckle or mole has popped up in the wrong place according to us, it pales in comparison to the whole package God created.

Comparisons. It is something we all do but to different degrees. We might be comparing ourselves to those very women who might be comparing themselves with us. When we compare ourselves with others, a few things can happen, like jealousy and depression. It can also bring along its sisters, pride, and arrogance. Comparisons divide and split the best of friends, delete the possibility of making new friends, and erase a multitude of positives in our lives. You must not worry what others think of you. No matter how many times I tell one of my daughters this, she seems to care all the more what others think. When we don't match up with the perfection society demands, our self-worth can shake and begin to crumble.

Our self-image is the way we think others see us. We may think others see us as fat, ugly, or socially inept, but that might be the farthest thing from reality. Self-esteem is what we believe of ourselves. If we feel like others do not truly like us, then our self-esteem can drop to dangerously low levels. When we do that thing called "compare and size up," it is reported we average a ninety-five percent return rate of negativity.[17] There is a belief that the brain cannot entertain two contradictory notions at the same time; eventually, one wins. If our self-talk begins churning up the grime from deep hurts, negatives will keep spewing out all over and will not allow the positives to proceed. Our negativity is like an open faucet. If we are not right with God, or listen to His Holy Spirit directing our paths, our thoughts will cause havoc and take us to a place we do not want to go.

When hurt by a friend, taken captive by inner thoughts, injured by self-pity or judged by others, low self-esteem sticks with us harder than body fat. These deep feelings affect us no matter how much we appear to have rock solid emotions. We sure know how to pull it off and look like we have it together. Some women have above average healthy physical bodies, but their self-esteem is wounded and hanging by threads. Their identity is stolen, and they do not realize who they truly are. This lie could have come from others, the enemy, or even themselves. Their low self-esteem encourages them to be physically supreme, so others will upgrade their thoughts about them, which is the typical conflict with comparison.

External beauty is fleeting. We are never going to have the fittest legs or core forever. There will always be someone more youthful with fewer wrinkles and better hair. The Bible says to focus on our inner self more than the external, but it does not say to totally ignore the external. 1 Peter 3:3 says that we should not let our adornment be merely outward, arranging the hair, wearing gold or putting on fine clothes as the focus; rather we should let the hidden person of our hearts show our real beauty. Inner beauty has no expiration date.

"We might be comparing ourselves to those very women who might be comparing themselves with us."

ARMOR ALERT: Who Am I in Christ?

1. **This invisible war can severely mess with the way we see ourselves physically. In the space below, write descriptive words that best define you or draw a self-portrait of your entire body. Please be as honest as possible.**

2. **In the Treasure Chest in the section: Who I Am in Christ, there is a list of various Scriptures telling us who God says we are. Say these verses audibly and claim them over your life.**

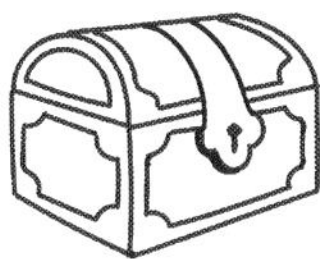

3. **Do you honestly believe who the Bible says you are in Christ?**

Testimony

I realized I was overweight when I was in second grade. After the birth of my second child, my weight had managed to climb to 260 and my cholesterol was at 238. At age 20, my OB told me that if I did not make a change in my life, I would automatically be placed on a cholesterol medication for the rest of my life. I knew I needed to make a change, not only for myself, but also for my family. I joined our local gym and started walking on the treadmill. There was a lot of positive encouragement there and I eventually found myself taking classes and meeting new friends, including Sarah.

Looking back, losing weight was the easy part. It has been the emotional ride I have been on since losing ninety pounds that has been the hard part. I worked out six to seven days a week and ate small portion sizes, cut sugars out, and would lose a pound here and there, but as soon as I would cheat, my weight would bounce back. I even ran a half-marathon and thought surely I would be able to lose the last 15 pounds. In reality, I was burning so many calories that I found myself craving more carbs. I had muscle cramps, pulled a hamstring, and my knees were starting to ache from running on the treadmill so much. I was not letting my body rest. If I missed a day of exercise I would feel so guilty. Not only that, but the scale also consumed me. I weighed myself morning and night every single day to make sure I was not gaining anything back.

After two years of this emotional juggling act, I realized how unhappy I was worrying about my weight constantly. It was adding stress to everyone. After finally coming to grips that I was never going to hit the normal weight, I am now wrapping my mind around contentment in my life. The Lord has blessed me with a great husband and four healthy children. I am learning that it is more important to be happy with the extra weight I carry, as long as I am healthy on the inside.

God has always been a part of my life, but I always thought that I had complete control over my life. To truly be happy, you have to rely on your faith in God. I am holding faith in the fact that He will help me maintain a HEALTHY weight for my body but balance a happy, healthy life that I can maintain. It is about a healthier lifestyle, not depriving myself of every indulgence out there, because that will just lead to more stress in life. With God's help, I am learning to be happy within my own skin while being the best mom and role model I can be and realizing that life is so much more important than what you see on the outside. What is on the inside is what truly counts!

Erin Engelbrecht
Donahue, Iowa

Before You Meet

The Pre-Evaluation Chart is a tool to help monitor your progress every two weeks. This week was all about your mental health. I trust you learned a few battle strategies on how to better arm yourself against mental assaults. Look through your underlined words in your Pre-Evaluation Chart using the words below. Then within your heart, monitor any progress.

Left side of chart: negative, mean, selfish, insecure, jealous, listening to poor reports, prideful, angry, entitled, unorganized, too busy, overwhelmed

Right side of chart: stable, solid, wise, secure, humble, sound-minded, positive, sober-minded, self-controlled, productive, driven, humble, scheduled, balanced, focused

Trainer Talk

Your physical activity should be on autopilot, or getting close to it. It may always be a challenge for some women to exercise. Exercise isn't at the top of the list for everyone—just like baking isn't on mine. I'm hoping your 2-Week Challenge is helping and not hindering your mental health. The point is to keep moving forward with some type of challenge—no matter how small. Ask God to help you and remember that you can do all things through Christ.

Look at your AP in the eyes when you meet next, and tell her that you are excited to spend eternity in heaven with her and what you think that will look like!

IT'S TIME TO MEET!

SECTION SEVEN

SWORD OF THE SPIRIT

This last section will tie together the entire Armor of God and your health. The first week focuses on the sword of the Spirit, which is the Word of God, and how this helps you be fully equipped in life—in and through the Holy Spirit. The second chapter brings back each piece of armor and summarizes how to apply it all through the help of the Holy Spirit. These two chapters are pivotal in this journey with a lot of application. For this reason, there are only three days of devotionals instead of four.

I am very proud of you for not exiting this journey early. I've witnessed many women who have given up too early on important goals. You have learned great biblical and practical tools that can help in years to come concerning your spiritual, physical, emotional, mental, and social health. I prayed that you would make the most of this last section, and do it with all strength, diligence, and vigor.

Be blessed and encouraged, my friend. You are an amazing woman who is beautifully and wonderfully made on the inside and out!

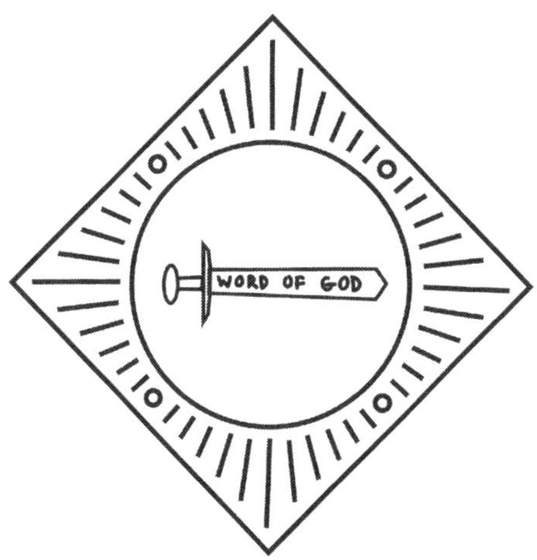

Week 13: Being Fully Equipped
Week 14: Arm Yourself with Whole Health

Health Challenge #6
2-Week Full Armor Challenge

Go back and look through all the challenges up to this date. Choose any you feel you need another shot at, need to continue with, or want to give another try. The last two weeks are going to focus on tying everything together.

1. **Health Challenge #1: 2-Week Nutrition Challenge**
2. **Health Challenge #2: 2-Week Emotional Challenge**
3. **Health Challenge #3: 2-Week Relationship Challenge**
4. **Health Challenge #4: 2-Week Stepping out in Faith Challenge**
5. **Health Challenge #5: 2-Week Mentally Strong Challenge**

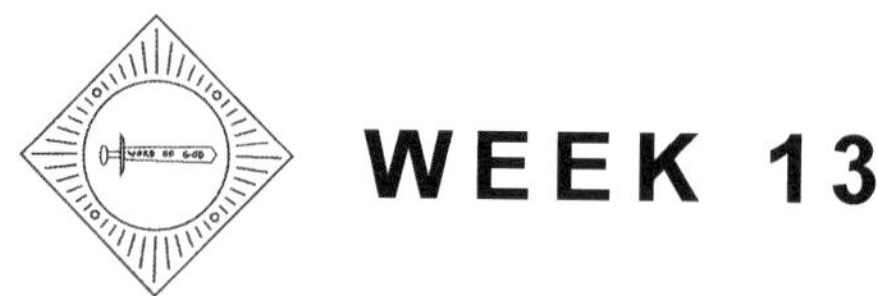

WEEK 13

BEING FULLY EQUIPPED

Week 13, Day 1
Sword of the Spirit

"And take the helmet of salvation, and the sword of the Spirit, which is the Word of God; praying always with all prayer and supplication in the Spirit, being watchful to this end with all perseverance and supplication for all the saints."
—Ephesians 6:17-18

A sword can demand, kill, destroy, protect, and claim victory. It is powerful but mainly in the physical sense. A great comparison is the Word of God and a double-edged sword (Hebrews 4:12), which provides conviction, rebuke, training, and cuts right to the heart. It sears the soul and spirit, joints and marrow, and judges the thoughts and attitudes of each of us. It is a supernatural fighting weapon—a sword used in the spirit realm. The Bible is the most influential living book in the world and is applicable in all its truths for us today. We are meant to use the Bible, the sword of the Spirit, not store it for safe-keeping or take it out only in emergency situations (the enemy would love that).

When something interferes and challenges the way people want to live, they can become irrational with justification. By our nature alone, we don't want to feel guilty or own up to our sin. We'd be happy to cover it up with lies or manipulation if left on our own. Thank the good Lord this is not the case for us all. Jesus has given us the Holy Spirit and the Word to convict, train, and help us with our unrighteousness. The Bible is truth and is very clear about what is right and wrong. This truth goes against our sin nature, which makes some want to even take it out of the government, schools, and churches.

We use a sword to fight physical battles and should use the Sword of the Spirit to fight spiritual ones. Jesus used Scripture in the desert to combat the garbage Satan threw against Him. Satan twisted the very words Jesus came to fulfill. He assaulted Jesus' weary body with false claims and mangled truths—none was with a natural weapon. Physical weapons are not useful in the spirit world. Jesus took Scripture and used it to make Satan flee. If you want your demons to retreat, submit yourself to God and pray using Scripture, like Jesus did (James 4:7). Allow God's Word to do the supernatural fighting; His Word will fight for you. Take the pressure off and give it all to God.

From Jesus' example, we know the enemy will try to use Scripture against us. But the enemy will twist it and make truth into a lie. He's so crafty at his art that if we don't know the real truth, we will fall into his trap—a major reason why it is imperative we know what the Bible truly says. Satan starts the lies and uses false teachers as his mouthpiece to proclaim them. If we spend a lot of time learning what the false truths are, we could easily become confused. Paul warns us and says to know the truth and flee from evil (2 Timothy 2:22). If you know the Bible, you do not need to spy in on the enemy's next move.

We must expose the lies and continue to speak the truth at all costs. Keep your hearts and minds tightly shut from false truths and teachings by engaging with the Sword of the Spirit (2 Peter 2). Always go back to the Scriptures for truth—be a fact checker. Just because someone looks like a sheep or a follower of Christ with education or eloquent speech does not mean they are. False teachers distract Christ-followers from obeying the truth of the Gospel. Teachers who take their congregation away from the truth of the Gospel are the false teachers depicted in 2 Peter. God has a strong warning for them: "To the law and to the testimony! If they do not speak according to this word, it is because there is no light in them" (Isaiah 8:20).

Even if a preacher says a particular sin is now permissible, such as being drunk with wine, the Bible is clear that it is wrong (Ephesians 5:18), the preacher is false in his teaching. He cannot choose individual practices and deem them justifiably okay because the current culture does. We can't follow part of the truth in the Bible and not all of it. I challenge you to double check what you hear in your services. It will not only keep your leaders accountable; it will keep you plugged into the Word of God.

It is never a pleasant experience to expose false teachers, but it is imperative to protect those younger in Christ, plus Christ commands it. Accepting differing religious options are not all spokes on a wheel leading to the same hub. Some religious beliefs lead to slavery and bondage, guilt and condemnation. Be obedient to God and worship where He leads you—not a new type of interpretation that sounds good (2 Timothy 4:3).

Pray and seek God with all your heart and lean on Him for strength, guidance, wisdom, and direction in your walk of faith. There are fantastic churches that have accountability and are fully proclaiming Christ with all vigor and vitality. If you are not part of a church like this, I challenge you to find one.

ARMOR ALERT: Going to Church?

Was your mind wandering while in church this past week? Just *being* in church does not mean you are earning brownie points with God. It is good spiritual discipline to go to church, but if you are not listening, or the words aren't processing in your brain, evaluate why you are there. We can be asleep on the inside yet perform all the motions on the outside, faking our faith to those around us.

1. **Are you taught truth at your place of worship? How do you know?**

2. **Explain if you have ever witnessed someone sharing false truth.**

3. **Go back to Week 1 and look over the commitment from Day 4. You were asked to memorize a verse. Can you say it for your AP/AG the next time you meet?**

4. **Meditate on your Scripture verse and pray. Use the ACTS below to help guide your prayer time if needed.**

ACTS
Acclamation—Proclaim how awesome He is.
Confession—Confess your sins and repent; get right with Him.
Thanksgiving—Thank Him for everything you can imagine.
Supplication—Lay your burdens for others and yourself at His feet.

Week 13, Day 2
Truth Alters Your Thinking

"...praying always with all prayer and supplication in the Spirit, being watchful to this end with all perseverance and supplication for all the saints—and for me, that utterance may be given to me, that I may open my mouth boldly to make known the mystery of the gospel, for which I am an ambassador in chains; that in it I may speak boldly, as I ought to speak."
—Ephesians 6:18-20

At times, I have to hear things more than once for them to really sink in. For this reason, I am recapping the second section of this book to challenge and see how much you remember.

Looking back on Section Two: Arm Yourself with Truth, Weeks 3 and 4 was dedicated to the truth of the Gospel and nutritional health. When there is ultimate truth present (the truth of Christ), our perspectives change, and we live our lives differently. It is like our daily interactions have a new approach with a deeper purpose. No longer do we focus and stress about things in the 21st-century. The attention shifts from our "I" and places it on others and God (the two greatest commandments).

Write down a few sentences from the titles below on what you remember most.

The daily titles for Week 3:

1. **Truth of the Gospel**—We arm ourselves by knowing the truth of the Gospel.

2. **Blenders of Truth**—We arm ourselves by recognizing half-truths.

3. **Don't Take the Bait**—We arm ourselves by renewing our minds with Scripture.

4. **Who's Leading Who?**—We arm ourselves by believing God's Word.

We dedicated Week 4 to our nutritional health. God wants us to thrive and live life as intended and to enjoy the earth, the different foods, and the many beautiful locations in which to eat. No matter our current physical state or location, we can still choose to eat healthy to the best of our abilities and resources. We do not have to be completely healthy gurus to fulfill God's assignments; being healthy just makes it a lot more enjoyable. Our minds would be cloudy without food for 40 days. My mind is cloudy after half a day without food. It is important to fuel our bodies correctly—think back to Goldilocks with not too much and not too little. Our body is the temple of the Holy Spirit. Just as we take care of our places of worship, our churches, we should likewise take extreme care of our tent, our bodies.

Record a few sentences below on what you remember most.

The daily titles for Week 4:

1. **Banking on Your Health**—We arm ourselves by investing in a plan.

2. **The Master Nutritionist**—We arm ourselves by following God's plan.

3. **Truth Behind Your Calories**—We arm ourselves by understanding God's calculations.

4. **What to Eat?**—We arm ourselves by sticking to the plan.

Problems can surface when we rarely prepare our food. When we eat out, the countless options of *smell-good* meals can overpower us. After a long stressful day, our taxed minds and bodies use the excuse that someone should handle this area for us—and we will pay top dollar for this luxury. After all, we have served everyone else all day. Our health is the greatest physical gift God created. We should take care of it with all our heart. Pray and ask God to help cravings when they come. Tell the "I" to leave when it wants to take over.

We learned that if we fail with physical activity and satisfy our body with poor nutrition, we won't get too far until we see repercussions. We can play the mental game with justification on why we cannot exercise or eat right. The "I" can make stress a justifying factor. I want to remind you, that you have the education, with practical plans and spiritual tools, to overcome internal health battles. You can stand in the victory that Christ is with you. Do not leave Him out of your health agenda. You can do more with Christ than without Him. Through Christ, you can do all things!

ARMOR ALERT: Healthy Recap

1. **Has your thinking been altered concerning God's truths?**

2. **Within these past 13 weeks, what one area have you accomplished in regards to your physical health?** (Celebrate with your AP/AG!)

3. **Which tools do you feel have helped you most with your nutrition?**

Week 13, Day 3

Righteousness Helps You Become Emotionally Fit

"Do not be wise in your own eyes; fear the Lord and depart from evil.
It will be health to your flesh and strength to your bones."
—Proverbs 3:7-8

When we are not right with God, it disturbs our spirit, which affects our emotions. For me, when I'm anything but righteous with God, it is like trying to swim upstream willingly with my arms tied behind my back. I know I need to get out of the water, dry off, and hang up my towel, but for some reason the "I" makes me keep swimming upstream alone. When I go on this way for too long, I feel as if I am drowning.

I'm most affected emotionally when God tests me, and I fail. After I fail a test, conviction follows. This is not guilt or shame but rather remorse that I let someone down that I love dearly. Nothing seems to go right because my emotions are irrational while in this disruptive state. I become a not-so-fun wife and mom. Stress begins to build walls of pride, and before I know it, I start putting up all kinds of wallpaper to hide things crumbling underneath. Once I've had enough fighting and failing with my paper swords, I remember I was the one who breached the relationship. Humility can be a costly lesson.

God loves to challenge us to create a better character and personal righteousness. He loves us dearly and desires the best for us. No matter what we do, He will not stop loving us (that is the best part about grace!). He is our life preserver and will save us. We just need to be humble and admit we are drowning.

We cannot suit up in God's Armor with the breastplate of righteousness by merely acting righteously or trying to do the right thing with the "I." Putting on righteousness goes beyond just being moral. A moralist has a list of ethical guidelines to follow to live a respectful life. We must surrender our heart and have a genuine desire to serve and honor Him because we love Him. Our morality should be a byproduct of following Christ. It is because of our love for Him that we have a profound moral commitment.

King David had a most impressive prayer as recorded in Psalm 25:4-5. He did not just pray for safety in battle; he asked God to keep him pure. In Psalm 141, he asked God to set a guard over his mouth, and to keep watch over the door of his lips, to not let his heart be drawn to what is evil or take part in wicked deeds. This prayer is very precise and all about the condition of His heart.

When our emotions start to get the best of us (especially with emotional eating, shopping, gossiping, and jealousy), we must ask God to make us pure. Purity produces righteousness in our hearts. It's the path to holiness. We can freely ask God to place a guard over our mouth, so evil won't slip in.

ARMOR ALERT: Emotional Recap

1. **Looking back at Week 5, you had an opportunity to look into your personal righteousness. What thoughts and experiences stuck with you most?**

   Week 5: Arm Yourself with Righteousness:

   1. **Righteousness**
   2. **Detox of the Heart**
   3. **Organizing Your Desires**
   4. **Commanded or Compelled?**

2. **What one or two thoughts will stick with you most from Week 6 concerning your emotional health?**

   Week 6: Arm Yourself with Emotional Health

   1. **Emotional Wars**
   2. **Emotional Jealousy**
   3. **Emotional Addictions**
   4. **Character Counts**
      (please keep Trainer Talk at the bottom of the page)

Trainer Talk

I want to bring something exciting to your attention. You have one more week until weigh-in day! Have you kept off that scale? Have you kept accountable with your weekly meetings with your AP?

IT'S TIME TO MEET!

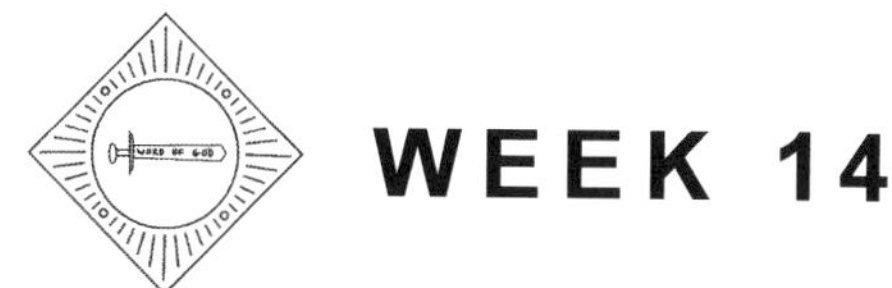

WEEK 14

ARM YOURSELF WITH WHOLE HEALTH

Week 14, Day 1

Peaceful People Are Social Heroes

"Mark the blameless man, and observe the upright; for the future of that man is peace."
—Psalm 37:37

If I react wildly to my husband for not closing the toilet lid after I sit and slip on in, and then find out it was my son's fault, I would be in deep water with my hubby. Quite a small battle, but it could grow ugly if I did not apologize correctly and immediately. Of course, there are larger battles I engage in that require humility at a deeper level. Apologizing to a family member for something small is easier than seeking restoration from lying or gossiping with a close friend.

Social heroes encourage instead of stir up strife. They bring peace, are not jealous or competitive, and don't talk poorly about other people. Gossip possesses an invisible intriguing pull to listen to the misfortune of others. Subsequently, there can be repercussions for merely listening. This antagonistic trap works very well on behalf of the enemy. The news of someone else in a compromised state makes us feel a little better about ourselves. There is also a misunderstanding that if we listen to gossip and don't share what we just heard, we aren't guilty of spreading it.

Every morning we can shod our feet with peace—we have that choice. We can ask God to fill us with the Holy Spirit to help us recognize when a test comes and to excel and obey in it. If we do this, we are more equipped to walk socially in peace. Our minds are in a better state, focused, and containing a right perspective. We are also more equipped to be a defender of others when trials come—like gossip. We could encounter huge social implications when shutting down gossip, especially if the one getting dumped on seems to deserve it. When we stick up for others, taking a possible step back on the social ladder won't matter as much to us. Our focus is on the bigger picture—our obedience to Christ. We can't allow the cares of this world to dictate if and when we should make peace with others. To prevail in our social health, we need to be at peace with God and led by the Holy Spirit.

It's easy to call people out on their sin (remember the plank in our eye and the speck in their eye?). We are social heroes when we do this in love and peace. Peace will open doors to other opportunities, such as sharing the Gospel. When we share our testimony with others, it's accepted better if peace is the center.

When I hear a bad report about someone else, I immediately think poorly of that person. That's my sinful nature within me. I don't want to feel that way, it just happens. I have learned those thoughts do not just go away either. When I see that person, those thoughts replay in my mind, even though I try not to have them. We all desire social acceptance and prominence. We want others to like us; it is in our nature. We want our name to stand on its own two legs. Help others through peace and build them up instead of tearing them down. We can't do this all too well on our own. We need the aid of the Holy Spirit, and through Him, you will be a witness for Christ and faultless in the eyes of others. We can all be a hero for Christ if we follow His standards.

ARMOR ALERT: Socially Inclined

1. **Section Four: Gospel of peace contained Chapters 7 and 8, which focused on spreading the Gospel and relationships through peace. With these titles listed below, record what you will take with you on your journey after completing this book.**

   Week 7—Arm Yourself with Peace

   Day 1: Gospel of Peace

   Day 2: Running Wildly

   Day 3: Actions are Louder than Megaphones

   Day 4: A Time to Share

   Week 8—Arm Yourself with Social Health

   Day 1: Faith Friends

   Day 2: Flourishing or Floundering Friendships

   Day 3: Muzzle Thy Mouth

   Day 4: Giving the Best in Each Relationship

2. **Think back to the 2-Week Social Challenge. Why did you choose this one?**

3. **Has the Holy Spirit led you to interact socially with others about Christ?** (Encourage, mentor, disciple, help, etc.)

Week 14, Day 2
With Faith Your Spiritual Health is Alive

"But you, beloved, building yourselves up on your most
holy faith, praying in the Holy Spirit."
—Jude 1:20

I have prayed for you to be individually challenged spiritually by the Lord. I have prayed for refreshed relationships with the Lord with increased Godly character. I trust He has shown you something new and exciting for your life through faith. Training for a marathon is hard yet so rewarding when crossing that finish line. Building your faith in Christ can likewise be hard when things around us seem like they are falling apart. When we spend time in His Word, we are slowly building our shields of faith, one verse at a time.

At the moment we finish our life race, and cross from earth to heaven, our finish line will be so much more than earning the trophy of being in heaven. Christ is the finisher of our faith journey (He's at the finish line) and will be with us after we cross that line into the heavenly realm—pure awesomeness. Knowledge of this alone can strengthen our spiritual health. Without it, there is no hope and nothing for which to strive. This fantastic grand prize should be beyond motivating for us to continue strong in our spiritual health.

There are many ways to increase our faith. We build our faith by praying with others in Jesus' name, sharing the Gospel, memorizing and reading Scripture, meditating on His Word, and spending time with Jesus—a recipe to protect us from the enemy and shield ourselves with faith in Christ. When we accept His unfailing love and forgiveness, step out and trust Him with our finances, or love others even when they are cruel to us, we are building our faith. When we ask God for divine intervention concerning our health, we place our trust in Him, and this too increases our confidence.

Our shields of faith strengthen with each step of confidence in Jesus, which make it that much harder for Satan's measly darts to penetrate. I have heard some people use the term "I'm on fire for Christ." This term can be confusing to others who aren't familiar with it. When we are on fire about something, we are one hundred percent involved. There is no question with onlookers; they can clearly see the passion in our cause. Our spiritual life takes it up a notch when our faith is strong. With our larger picture perspective and our all-in mentality, it should appear we are on fire for God. Our spiritual life should be alive and thriving, always growing and never stagnant in our faith.

ARMOR ALERT: Building?

This is an important Armor Alert today. Please record how you have built your faith these past few weeks, and then make it a point to share the answers with your AP when you meet next.

Week 14, Day 3
Salvation Makes You Mentally Savvy

"All Scripture is given by inspiration of God, and is profitable for doctrine, for reproof, for correction, for instruction in righteousness, that the man of God may be complete, thoroughly equipped for every good work."
—2 Timothy 3:16-17

Do you still catch yourself arguing inside your mind with that little tiny devil and angel sitting on either shoulder? The antagonist will be here for a while, but the good news is we now have a plan of action to combat him.

When I ask strangers about Jesus, they can reply, "I'm good." I then question why they think they are good. They tell me they don't want to hear about religion. I peacefully tell them there is nothing religious about Jesus. He came to save us from it, and the people who killed Him were the religious ones (the Pharisees). Religion blinded them from Jesus. Then I tell them they are not good without Christ, and in fact, they would be good with Him.

I'm shocked that many people do not know much about Jesus. Most are willing to listen once I prove it's not a religious matter, rather, a relationship. I ask the Holy Spirit to take my mind out of the process and make my heart the center so my conversations focus on His leading. Witnessing isn't always easy. I'm still learning to listen to the Holy Spirit's promptings to go do something. I think I will always be learning.

Some reject Christ because they think they have to live by stuffy codes and rules and do all these things to please Him. If you know God, it is quite the opposite. The more I know Him, the more freedom I have. I have more sustaining peace in my mind, which makes me want to please God even more. It's like my mind thinks clearer and I'm more mentally savvy.

Are you truly committed to Christ with your whole heart and mind? The enemy has plans to blockade your thoughts, but you have weapons to win and conquer him. Say and believe the Scripture that any weapon formed against you will not prosper (Isaiah 54:17). Claim the Scripture and trust God, if we meditate on His Word, whatever we do will prosper (Joshua 1:8).

Meditating is different than studying. When we meditate, we take the time to ponder. We process and think about how we could apply and grow. God says when we meditate on His Word, three things will happen—we will bear fruit, we will prosper in whatever we do, and it will cause us to understand the Word of God. Another step toward Godly wisdom will help foster holiness.

ARMOR ALERT: Meditation

You have arrived at your last Armor Alert. Take time with this one. There is no rush.

Think about Weeks 11 and 12 concerning your salvation and mental health. Record some thoughts on how these two weeks connected with you and any applications.

Testimony

The Sword of the Spirit is the Word of God (Ephesians 6:17). The Bible teaches that Jesus delegated His authority to His followers. To walk in that authority, His Word must abide (or live) on the inside of us (John 15:7), and start coming out of our mouths—we being fully convinced the Lord Himself will perform His Word (Romans 4:20-21).

In one year, I got two urinary tract infections (UTI). The first I could believe for a speedy recovery using the physician's prescription. That's what happened! My symptoms left sooner than the physician had predicted. I had been building up an arsenal of God's healing promises in my heart, plus I had the desire to overcome sickness as Jesus did. Jesus is aggressively opposed to sickness. What's more, He has bought our bodies (1 Corinthians 6:20).

Therefore, I resist sickness being on God's property, my body! It may have taken 10 to 14 days before all symptoms of the UTI disappeared, but the sword of the Spirit in praise, authority, and thanksgiving prevailed!

And every victory you obtain by faith just gets sweeter and sweeter in your walk with Jesus.

Anna Marie Percuoco
Long Grove, IA

The Post-Test: A Snapshot of Your Overall Health

Now that you have learned new insight into a healthier lifestyle look at the Post-Evaluation chart on the following page. What an opportunity to see growth from the first time you took this test. Take a few honest minutes to reflect on your current health. Then, answer the questions below.

1. **Which area do you feel is your strongest concerning your health today?**
2. **In which area have you grown the most over these past 14 weeks?**
3. **What is your biggest takeaway from this entire journey?**
4. **Compare the results of your Pre-Evaluation Chart with your new results. Comment in the space below on any differences or similarities. Share this with your AP when you meet next.**

Finish the question: I am ...

Pre-Evaluation Chart

lazy, over/under weight, sporadic with exercise, negative, sickly, always dieting, too busy, lacking priorities, making excuses, unmotivated	**Physical Health** Week 2 _______ %	motivated, very routine, energized, driven, dedicated, a planner, fit, strong, healthy, active, consistent, comfortable exercising, excited about workouts
unscheduled, a meal-skipper, addicted, unplanned, apathetic, unhealthy, a binge eater, uncontrolled, gluttonous, obese, uneducated, craving	**Nutritional Health** Week 4 _______ %	scheduled, controlled, healthy, aware, confident, not addicted, committed, sustainable, planned, educated, not craving
sad, uncontrolled, weary, worn, jealous, judgmental, angry, depressed, unstable, closed-off, unrighteous in anger, selfish, entitled, toxic, unholy, afraid, shameful	**Emotional Health** Week 6 _______ %	happy, confident, stable, joyful, controlled, even tempered, peaceful, easy going, forgiving, a goal-setter, courageous, positive, obedient, building character
unfriendly, uncommitted, closed, wounded, a gossiper, a liar, a slanderer, Miss. attitude, flighty, aloof, draining on others, a manipulator, pressuring others	**Social Health** Week 8 _______ %	keeper of friendships, open, loving, available, a listener, thinking of others, serving others, tender-hearted, accepting, patient, honest
unsure of afterlife, unthankful, unloving, not giving, not witnessing, not professing truth, fake, closed, scared, unholy, not cleaving to God	**Spiritual Health** Week 10 _______ %	saved, peaceful, hopeful, faithful, truthful, righteous, meek, humble, loving, assured, holy, witnessing, forgiving, praying, listening
negative, mean, selfish, insecure, jealous, listening to poor reports, prideful, angry, entitled, unorganized, too busy, overwhelmed	**Mental Health** Week 12 _______ %	stable, solid, wise, secure, humble, sound-minded, positive, sober-minded, self-controlled, productive, driven, humble, scheduled, balanced, focused
Unbalanced physically, nutritionally, emotionally, socially, spiritually, and mentally unhealthy	**Overall Health** Week 14 _______ %	**Balanced** physically, nutritionally, emotionally, socially, spiritually, and mentally healthy

Before You Meet
Weigh Day Is Here

You have finally arrived at this ending point in your journey. Did you honestly wait to jump on that scale until today? Some of you are excited, and others are dreading to see those numbers.

Have you arrived at the point where your scale does not matter? It is just a number. How healthy you are on the inside and how your clothes feel and fit are your indicators.

The scale reflects the whole picture—how much your water, bones, muscles, body fat, hair, skin, organs, and blood all weigh. Fat is not the only thing we gain or lose when we step on a scale to measure progress. In certain workouts we build muscle, lose fat, and have different intakes of fluids which have significance when stepping on the scale. Another important fact to consider when weighing yourself, sometimes there is no apparent numeric progress—with bloating and water retention, when muscle-gain and fat-loss cancel each other out, or metabolism ups and downs.

It's time to weigh in!

1. **My new current weight is: ______________** (Remember it is not about weight but about how you feel and look in your clothes.)

2. **Are my clothes feeling looser?**

3. **Do I feel healthier?**

4. **Do I see progress according to God's standards?**

5. **Am I trying my hardest and really following the plan?**

**Reminder: You should not see more than a two-pound weight loss per week for healthy, efficient living.*

Share your results with your AP/AG.

IT'S TIME TO MEET!
(but hopefully not for the last time)

CONGRATULATIONS!

May your journey never stop, but prosper with all blessings from above. I am so very proud of you!

"I have competed well. I have finished the race. I have kept the faith."
—2 Timothy 4:7

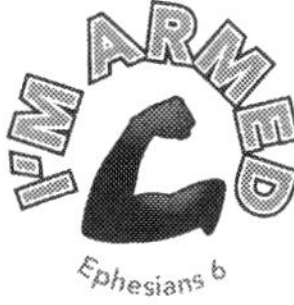

Because spiritual and physical battles will still rage on, we must always remember to keep ourselves ready and armed with God's Armor. Go to fullarmorfitness.com and get an Arm Yourself decal. Place it somewhere to remind you of your 14-Week journey and how you can overcome anything with Christ as your Commander.

I would love your feedback about your personal journey.
Email or leave a comment through my website, fullarmorfitness.com.

TREASURE CHEST

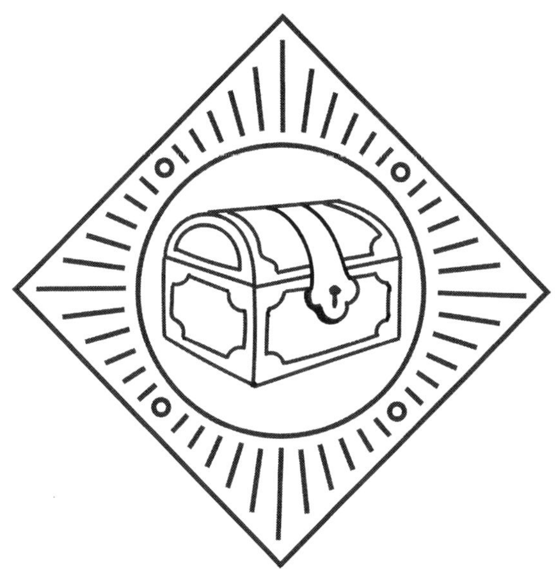

TREASURE CHEST INDEX

1. Surrender 226
2. Scriptures to Combat Doubt & Fear 229
3. Who I Am in Christ 230
4. Exercise Training Programs 231
    a. Step 1: Simple Planning 231
    b. Step 2: God's Fitness Tools 232
        i. Exercise Lingo & Frequency 232
        ii. Muscle & Cardiovascular Tools 233
        iii. God's Exercise Rules 233
        iv. What Cardio Intensity Is Right for Me? 234
        v. Find Your Estimated Target Heart Rate (THR) 234
        vi. Find Your Resting Heart Rate (RHR) 235
        vii. The Skinny Behind Calories 235
        viii. Styles of Training 236
        ix. Suggested Exercise Output 237
5. Step 3: Choose Your Level of Fitness 239
    a. Level 1 Program Option 240
    b. Level 2 Program Option 241
    c. Level 3 Program Option 242
    d. Exercise Plans 243
        i. 4-Minute Rounds 243
        ii. Boot Camp Circuit 244
        iii. Bottoms Up Circuit 1 245
        iv. Building Strength 246
        v. Burst Training 247
        vi. Butts & Guts 248
        vii. Core Circuits 249
        viii. Countdown 250
        ix. Double Trouble 251
        x. Down & Back 252
        xi. HIT Countdown 253
        xii. Increase Cardio & Speed 254
        xiii. Just Counting Steps 255
        xiv. Musical Core 256
        xv. Ninja Cardio Circuit 257
        xvi. Scorpion Sting 258
        xvii. Simply Moving 259
        xviii. Stretcher Prepper Plan 260
        xix. Take A Chance 261
        xx. Undie 500 262
        xxi. Upper Body Plans 263

xxii. You Choose Cardio 264

6. Meal Planning 287
   a. Meal Planning Step 1: Identify Your Real Consumption 287
      i. Meal Plan Levels 287
      ii. Cheat Sheet – Sarah's Basic Foods 288
   b. Meal Planning Step 2: Get A Grip on the Food Label 289
   c. Meal Planning Step 3: Identify Your Caloric Goals 290
      i. Breaking Down Your Calories 290
   d. Meal Planning Step 4: Choosing Wisely 292
   e. Meal Planning Step 5: Putting It Together – Simply 296
      i. Sample Blank Meal Plans 296
      ii. Every Day Meal Plans 299
      iii. Gluten & Dairy Free Meal Plans 301
      iv. Gluten Free Meal Plans 303
      v. Dairy Free Meal Plans 305
      vi. Lose Weight Meal Plans 307
      vii. Quick Tips on When to Eat 309
   f. Fit Recipes 310
      i. Fit Breakfasts 310
      ii. Fit Lunches 312
      iii. Fit Dinners 314
      iv. Snappy Side Dishes 317
      v. Healthy Desserts 318
      vi. Simple Snack List 319
   g. Dinner Planning Tips 321

SURRENDER

I have had friends who sat in church services for years and heard the Gospel but never really understood the full truth of it. They could not tell me anything more than the nativity scene. The meat of the Gospel is the why behind it. When we understand why we need to surrender to Christ, it is a whole new amazing and freeing life—in this life and in the one to follow.

When I think of the word "surrender," a few things come to mind. I think of someone holding up and waving a white flag showing they are lost, or I imagine a battle scene with someone waving their hands to show they are giving up, or I think of someone realizing they just cannot keep doing what they are doing, breaking down and asking for intervention. These three examples all demonstrate the reason we need to surrender to Christ. We are lost and can't win the death battle on our own, and we can't save ourselves from certain problems.

When one of my relationships is broken or strained, it hurts deeply, emotionally, and mentally. It affects more than I think. If I am not proactive about fixing it, I begin to churn it over and over in my heart with negativity, bitterness, or pride. I have a choice to intentionally mend a strained relationship or be prideful and push off fixing it. If we are willing to fix it, and surrender this relationship to God, He will heal and forgive us. This type of submission will help us become clean with God, but we still have other areas to yield. It's not just about surrendering our problems.

Romans 3:23 says we all have fallen short of the glory of God. Ephesians 2:5 tells us we are dead in our sins. If we died apart from God, we would be separated from Him forever (and forever is a super long time). God is holy and spiritually clean, but man is sinful and spiritually unclean. Just as a person cannot tolerate being by a dead animal carcass that is decaying and stinks, God cannot be near His creation when it is filthy and tainted with sin. The result of sin is clear—it made a barrier between God and man.

This barrier is such a large chasm; man's efforts cannot make a bridge. Something supernatural has to provide a way because humans are incapable. We cannot get there with physical means like money. In fact, our money does not buy us anything spiritual, including forgiveness. Tithing or giving more to the church has no bearing on being forgiven from sin and able to reach God. It does not matter if we go to church, obey, try to be moral, or volunteer at the soup kitchen. It is like fighting a ghost with an iron sword. We cannot fight the spiritual with natural means any more than we can erase sin with our pocketbooks or our good deeds.

In Isaiah 64:6, we read that we are like an unclean thing, and all our righteousness is as filthy rags. To attempt to wash away our own sin is like trying to clean a dirty face with a greasy rag. We cannot *do* anything in our own power to erase our sin and cross the barrier that separates us from God.

Our inability to be righteous is why it is so important to understand the Gospel. Once we truly realize we are lost and doomed without God due to our sin, our white "surrender" flag should wave so big everyone around us would see it. I would rather be with Jesus than dying without hope of an eternity with Him.

God is one hundred percent righteous and just. He knew we could not amend the barrier, and cross the chasm that separates us from Him, all by our human self. This is why He provided a cure, a means to heal us from our sin, and restore our relationship—the Gospel. The Gospel demonstrates grace. Grace is given to us and will never be stolen. Grace can't be earned and can't be lost, He loves us unconditionally (this is *why* the Gospel is called the Good News). There are over 160 verses in the New Testament that declare the only condition for receiving grace and eternal life is faith in Jesus Christ.

Jesus was born to a virgin (miracle) and lived a perfect life without sin (divine). He died a sacrificial death to pay the penalty for our sin that we could not pay ourselves because only someone without sin could pay the penalty for sin. Death could not hold Him in the grave because He is God (divine). He came back to life to tell us about it (miracle) and ascended to heaven, where He now sits at the right hand of God (see the book of John in the Bible). This is the elementary Gospel. It is to the point and makes sense. It is interesting and intriguing, yet begs for more. That is because the Gospel demands more than hearing alone. It requires a response.

Jesus came and sacrificed Himself while we were still sinners (Romans 5:8). He came to us while we were broken, and died for us (so we would not have to die). By doing this, Jesus, who knew no sin, became the substitute and sacrificed Himself so we could be restored with God—and cross the barrier to Him (2 Corinthians 5:21).

Christ's death paid in full our debt. Anyone who accepts Christ does not have to fear God's wrath or judgment. John 19:30 states, "When Jesus therefore received the vinegar on the cross He said, "it is finished," and He bowed His head and gave up His spirit." The phrase "it is finished" was an expression used in Rome in that time when a debt was paid in full. Jesus was telling everyone He completed the final payment for sin (Colossians 2:13-14).

To forgive sin, God righteously had to condemn sin in another—His son Jesus. This shows that forgiveness is not cheap. It is the most priceless currency ever.

God requires that we believe (trust) in Jesus. We must give up the "I" in order to surrender to Him. Beware, the "I" will try to muddy the waters and make excuses for sin. It plays tricks on us and presents doubt, fear, unbelief, and makes us feel that Jesus is implausible, unreliable, and unattainable. It makes the Gospel seem unattractive and cheap.

We cannot fake it and make it with God. He knows our hearts and if we are truthful with our surrender to Him. We will fail at this relationship with Him unless we truly repent. He promises to forgive us. We must surrender our entire lives continually to Christ. We must renew our minds with prayer daily (sometimes I have to hourly), read Scripture, go to church, and have accountability partners to keep us growing continually in our relationship with Christ.

The most personal decision you will ever make is with Christ. Tell Him your feelings and hand over your true allegiance. Ask Him to forgive you and make you clean. Communicate with Him now. He always has an open door. Surrendering all will bring more freedom and abundant living than you could ever imagine.

SCRIPTURES TO COMBAT DOUBT & FEAR

1. "Behold, I have given you authority to tread on serpents and scorpions, and over all the power of the enemy, and nothing shall hurt you" (Luke 10:19, ESV).
2. "For we know that if the tent that is our earthly home is destroyed, we have a building from God, a house not made with hands, eternal in the heavens" (2 Corinthians 5:1, ESV).
3. "Seek the Lord and his strength; seek his presence continually" (Psalm 105:4, ESV).
4. "The Lord upholds all who are falling and raises up all who are bowed down" (Psalm 145:14, ESV).
5. "Even youths shall faint and be weary, and young men shall fall exhausted; but they who wait for the Lord shall renew their strength; they shall mount up with wings like eagles; they shall run and not be weary; they shall walk and not faint" (Isaiah 40:30-31, ESV).
6. "You have given me the shield of your salvation, and your right hand supported me, and your gentleness made me great. (Psalm 18:35, ESV).
7. "He rescued me from my strong enemy and from those who hated me, for they were too mighty for me" (Psalm 18:17, ESV).
8. "Be strong, and let your heart take courage, all you who wait for the Lord" (Psalm 31:24, ESV).
9. "But he said to me, "My grace is sufficient for you, for my power is made perfect in weakness." Therefore I will boast all the more gladly of my weaknesses, so that the power of Christ may rest upon me" (2 Corinthians 12:9, ESV).
10. "And he hath said unto me, My grace is sufficient for thee: for my power is made perfect in weakness. Most gladly therefore will I rather glory in my weaknesses, that the power of Christ may rest upon me" (2 Corinthians 12:9, ESV).
11. "So also is the resurrection of the dead. It is sown in corruption; it is raised in incorruption: it is sown in dishonor; it is raised in glory: it is sown in weakness; it is raised in power: it is sown a natural body; it is raised a spiritual body. If there is a natural body, there is also a spiritual body" (1 Corinthians 15:42-44, ESV).
12. "I can do all things through him who strengthens me" (Philippians 4:13, ESV).

WHO I AM IN CHRIST

1. I am faithful. (Ephesians 1:1)
2. I am God's child. (John 1:12)
3. I have been justified. (Romans 5:1)
4. I am Christ's friend. (John 15:15)
5. I am assured all things work together for good. (Romans 8:28)
6. I have been established, anointed and sealed by God. (2 Corinthians 1:21-22)
7. I am a citizen of heaven. (Philippians 3:20)
8. I have not been given a spirit of fear, but of power, love and self-discipline. (2 Timothy 1:7)
9. I am born of God and the evil one cannot touch me. (1 John 5:18)
10. I am blessed in the heavenly realms with every spiritual blessing. (Ephesians 1:3)
11. I was chosen before the creation of the world. (Ephesians 1:4, 11)
12. I am holy and blameless. (Ephesians 1:4)
13. I have redemption. (Ephesians 1:8)
14. I am forgiven. (Ephesians 1:8; Colossians 1:14)
15. I have purpose. (Ephesians 1:9, 3:11)
16. I have hope. (Ephesians 1:12)
17. I am salt and light of the earth. (Matthew 5:13-14)
18. I have been chosen and God desires me to bear fruit. (John 15:1, 5)
19. I am a personal witness of Jesus Christ. (Acts 1:8)
20. I am alive with Christ. (Ephesians 2:5)
21. I have peace. (Ephesians 2:14)
22. I have access to the Father. (Ephesians 2:18)
23. I am secure. (Ephesians 2:20)
24. I can be humble, gentle, patient, and lovingly tolerant of others. (Ephesians 4:2)
25. I can mature spiritually. (Ephesians 4:15)
26. I can be certain of God's truths and the lifestyle to which He has called me. (Ephesians 4:17)
27. I can have a new attitude and a new lifestyle. (Ephesians 4:21-32)
28. I can forgive others. (Ephesians 4:32)
29. I am a light to others and can exhibit goodness, righteousness, and truth. (Ephesians 5:8-9)
30. I do not have to always have my own agenda. (Ephesians 5:21)

EXERCISE TRAINING PROGRAMS

STEP 1: SIMPLE PLANNING

Below is a sample of how to organize your exercise. However you schedule it, just make sure it is balanced and sustainable. Over-exercising in your younger years can lead to prolonged and chronic issues as you age. One of my favorite sayings when it comes to exercise—"Just because you can doesn't mean you should." Fill in the blanks on this chart.

Example Training Plan			
Sample Week	**Training & Where**	**With Who?**	**Time of Day**
Sunday	Rest		
Monday	Burst & Strength Training — at gym		8:30am-9:30am
Tuesday	Deep Stretching — at home		9:15am-10am
* Wednesday	Strength Training — at gym Running — outside	Nick	8:30am-9:30am 8pm-8:30pm
Thursday	Rest (stretching)		
Friday	Cardio Fitness class	Elisa	8:30am-9:30am
Saturday	Speed Walking	Marianna	7am-8am
Your Training Plan	**Training & Where**	**With Who?**	**Time of Day**
Sunday			
Monday			
Tuesday			
Wednesday			
Thursday			
Friday			
Saturday			
Optional Double Day?			

STEP 2: GOD'S FITNESS TOOLS

Below, you will find exercise terms and training guidelines that are extremely helpful when performing an exercise program. Think of this as your personal trainer. This section explains the 'why' behind what we are doing—with safety guidelines for effective training. It includes many styles of training and their benefits, the background of how you burn calories more efficiently, how to find your target heart, and much more.

Exercise Lingo & Frequency

Sets: The number of 1 complete repetition cycle. Repeating an exercise 10 times (reps) for example equals 1 set. A set can be any number of reps.

Reps: (short for repetition) The number of times you repeat the same exercise in a row. Reps can be any length in repetition.

Strength Training: Conditioning the muscles with weight and resistance training to improve muscle and bone density with overall strength. If these following plans seem confusing, or if you are unsure of the details, seek out a personal trainer for help. If you cannot afford a trainer, join fitness classes. You can learn the basics of lifting in a group fitness class with a certified instructor. Aim to perform weight lifting 2-4 days per week with a 48-hour rest before exercising the same muscle groups again.

Sample Lifting Schedules:

Beginner-Intermediate—lift 2 to 4 days per week. Lift every other day. Perform 1-2 sets of 8 repetitions (1x8 or 2x8).

Intermediate-Advanced—lift 5 to 6 days per week. Alternate days between the upper and lower body. Alternate days from pulling to pushing exercises. Perform 3 sets of 8 repetitions (3x8) or 4 sets of 6 (4x6).

More Bulk: If you desire to add bulk or have a stronger looking build, add more weight and perform fewer reps. You should come to a point in the lift when you feel a harder struggle in the exercise once you hit around 4 to 8 reps. If you don't, consider adding more weight.

More Tone & Cut: If you desire to add lean and slender muscle or a less bulky look, lessen the weight and perform more reps. Alternate days between the upper and lower body. Alternate days between pulling and pushing exercises. Perform 2 sets of 20 reps (2x20) or 2 sets of 30 reps (2x30).

I love this verse. It reminds me that it's okay for women to be strong. "She girds herself with strength; she exerts her arms with vigor" (Proverbs 31:17).

Muscle & Cardiovascular Tools

Our hearts and lungs operate differently than the muscles wrapped around our bones. They are involuntary and used continuously, even if just sitting in the chair. These are the gals that require constant energy and calories to make us survive (BMR—calories burned by involuntary function). These muscles and processes work extra hard when we exercise, or take a heavy load of laundry up those stairs. Exercise will improve these involuntary muscles, so when we are at rest, they will work all the more efficiently.

Note that we can stop cardio activity for about two weeks before it begins to reverse in progress.

If we want to lose body fat, we will have to raise our heart rate (HR—the rate our blood pumps in and out of our heart) three to five times per week. The higher the intensity, the longer the run or the different frequencies (hi/low) we perform exercises will all help us burn fat.

The muscles wrapped around our bones work differently than our involuntary ones, the heart, and lungs. These gals need movement to maintain muscle or grow in strength.

"God made our bodies and knows all the in and outs, obviously, so do not skimp on His guidelines."

God did not create women in general as strong as men physically—that was His choice. It doesn't mean we aren't as strong in other areas. I think I would win the endurance and pain test giving birth to children over my husband. Men are made differently and can attain larger growth in their muscles due to their hormones. If we were to take these same hormones, we could bulk with outstanding results.

Some women want to look bulky and thick. Some want to look thin. Some just want to be healthy and do not care what their muscles even look like. It is your choice with the desired outcome, but please consider adding some weight to your workouts. It will increase your bone density, lean muscle mass, and add many more benefits to make you healthier overall.

**Please remember to talk to your physician about your cardiac output before engaging in any exercise, especially if you are pregnant, have a heart condition, metabolic disease, are on medication, or have high blood pressure.*

God's Exercise Rules

God will not make us work out and will not make us stick to this program. That choice is ours individually. We will personally make the decision to stick with our commitments or not. Even though God will not make us do certain things, He does give guidelines when we choose to engage in some of them, like exercise. For this reason, God created a rule our bodies need to follow. It is one of those natural laws.

 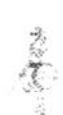

48-72 Hour Muscle Rule: If we exercise a particular muscle group, like our biceps, they need to rest and restore themselves before they are extended again. If you worked your biceps on Monday, you should wait until Wednesday (48 hours) to lift. Let's say Wednesday you are busy and could not exercise. Good news—you have until Thursday (72 hours) to work out again before cessation begins (regression). Sometimes the spirit is willing, but the flesh is weak. Many days I do not want to exercise, but I know I need to. We can be like Jesus and ask God to give our flesh strength to continue with our plan.

What Cardio Intensity Is Right for Me?

Generally speaking, those who already exercise know their limits. If you do not know how hard to push yourself, or are new to exercise, it is imperative you seek medical advice or see a fitness expert before engaging in cardiovascular activity. There are guidelines all fitness providers must follow, and these guidelines help keep everyone safe and healthy.

If you have a heart issue, high blood pressure, older than 65 years old, completely new to exercise, pregnant, or should not elevate your heart rate because of medicines you are taking, obtain clearance from your physician. Three questions you should consider asking your Physician; how high should you get your heart rate, how long should you exercise your heart, and with what intensity.

For example, some healthy looking individuals should not perform interval training because it stresses their heart. Just like some people with metabolic issues that should not be on a treadmill for an hour. Their blood sugar could get too low. If you are new to exercise, please pay special attention to your heart rate during workouts and speak to your overseeing expert.

If you are sixty-five or older, there is no reason to max out your heart rate with exercise. If you are taking medication to lower your blood pressure, it is dangerous to make your heart rate high during exercise. The most important guideline to follow is you—and your physician. Listen to your body. Please do not neglect to talk to your physician if you are unsure about any exercise program.

Find Your Estimated Target Heart Rate (THR)

Are you working too hard, too little, or just enough? For the general population, if you are trying to lose weight and exercise using a treadmill, you should not have enough gusto in your lungs to be able to sing at the same time—you would not be working hard enough to lose weight. If exercising at 50% intensity, one would need to work out longer to achieve results as someone exercising at 85% intensity.

This below formula is for the general population, those not taking any medications, or those without existing health conditions.

Maximum Heart Rate (MHR) Formula

Women: 220 ____________ (age) = ____________ MHR

Target Heart Rate (THR) Formula

MHR x .50 = ____________

MHR x .85 = ____________

My THR Zone is between: ____________ - ____________

The above equation is estimation for cross-training, aerobics, running, and land exercises. If you are biking, subtract 5 beats per minute. If you are swimming, subtract up to 10 beats per minute.

For the first few weeks when you begin any training program, you should strive to the lower end of your target heart rate zone, 50%-60%. Once comfortable, slowly build your efforts towards 70% to 85%—if needed and able.

Find Your Resting Heart Rate (RHR)

Your resting heart rate lends significant clues to a healthy heart. If your heart beats higher or lower than average when at rest, consider seeing your physician about possible issues. An average resting heart rate can be anywhere between 60-100 beats per minute according to the US Department of Health and Human Services.

For three days in a row, take your heart rate for one full minute at either of the two times suggested below. Once you have all three results, take the average.

1. When you first wake up, before you get out of bed.
2. After you have sat for 20 full minutes doing nothing (like reading or watching TV).

The Skinny Behind Calories

Calculating how many calories you dropped in a fitness class or after a 10-mile run is hard to figure out without certain tools, such as a heart rate monitor. We spend so much money on toys and trinkets that tell how many steps we took or calories we burned. These tools, like anything else, can help or hinder. I used to keep track of every calorie I burned—which was a big mistake. My problem was that when I did not burn enough calories, I became frustrated. This led me to train harder so I could burn more calories and hit my goal. This is an easy recipe for addiction. It can easily consume and overpower our focus.

If we perform interval-based exercises such as burst training, our caloric burn will be much higher *after* we workout, and our calorie counter will not show this during exercise or after we take the calorie counter off. When we participate in intervals, our heart rate gets very high and then recovers. The overall caloric burn won't match if we compare it to traditional calorie-burning based routines.

The incredible advantage of intervals is that we burn more calories during rest and recovery in the following days. The heart rate monitor only reads each heartbeat and calculates those beats into calories burned. When we rest during an interval, it will tell us we are not burning as many calories, but we are burning fat as our bodies recover and repair. Great tool, but it does not work for every type of exercise.

If you want to track your burned calories when performing interval-based exercises, estimate. Sometimes this process will just take time to figure out. If you are working hard, following your body's cues, and enjoying the fact that you are sticking to it, then this in itself is enough to focus on. If you want to find out how many calories you are burning, which in all honesty can be fun at times, there are a few methods. Below are just the easiest two.

Your first option is to buy a heart rate monitor that tells how many calories you burned. This is important because some do not record calories burned, they just keep track of your pulse. Once you purchase it, take about five minutes to plug in your weight, height, age, target heart rate zone, and resting heart rate (these numbers are found under God's Exercise Rules). I suggest getting an HRM with a chest strap.

Another option is to use your treadmill or elliptical or stationary bike to help keep track of calories burned if it has a heart rate monitor system. Not all machines have this option. You must plug in your weight and age beforehand for a suggested caloric burn. If you do not type in your age and weight, the machine will give a range of calories burned based off a universal weight and age.

Styles of Training

Being active in a gym or fitness center provides a fantastic social outlet, which I highly recommend. But don't worry, I totally understand that a public workout facility can be super intimidating. Plus, not everyone has access. It is healthy socially to be in public at times, but fine to be in seclusion as well. I suggest you mix it up a little for your emotional and social health. The below list reflects training styles in order, starting at the beginning level. Everyone has a preferred style; this is the joy in experimenting.

Balance we can increase balance at any age. We shouldn't push this off until later in life. It will aid in walking, squatting, performing countless exercises, and help in overall well-being. We use balance more than we realize in our everyday living. Plus, it aids in core strength. Generally speaking, the better our balance, the stronger our core.

Stretching is elongating our muscles with targeted breathing for a certain amount of time. Stretching is one the most versatile and essential styles of exercise in a training program, yet it gets the least amount of attention. Some studies show the average person should devote 50% of their fitness to stretching, 25% to resistance, and 25% to cardio. We should never bounce or force a muscle past the threshold of pain. The lower the force of stretching, the greater the permanent lengthening of the muscle. We can stretch at about 50% longer than a usual resting length.[18]

Core Work can be combined with many other exercises. If we perform a plank, we are using our stomach, the sides of our stomach, our back as well as our upper body to maintain that plank. We will focus on our complete core (not just the tummy) by using abdominal muscles, obliques, and back.

Steady Cardio is a set pace for a given amount of time, usually 30-45 minutes or a set number of miles or kilometers. This form of training is good, but not for everyday health by itself. Other styles of exercise must be included in your program, such as strength training and stretching.

Strength Training is the use of resistance on your body as you increase or maintain strength. Lifting weights or heavy objects, using resistance tubes, bands or your own body weight are examples. There are countless forms of strength training with different weights, reps, sets, and styles.

Interval Training and Plyometrics are performed with any high/low combination—getting our heart rate high and then low. *If you are pregnant or have any heart issues, please see your physician before engaging in intense cardio training.

Burst Training is a form of interval training with a very hard cardio output with twice the length of recovery time. The formula is easy—60 seconds of intense cardio followed by 120 seconds of recovery, repeated 4 to 5 full rotations of time. The benefit of burst training is that this style burns more fat after you are finished, for up to 48 hours in some cases. Remember we compared a sprinter and a long distance participant. A sprinter participates in burst training. They run around the track as hard and fast as possible, and they fully and completely rest before they do it again.

High-Intensity Training is engaging in bouts of higher intensity physical exercise with or without giving the body as much rest in between exercises. Your recovery time can vary between exercises or sets of exercises. For instance: Perform 60 jumping jacks and immediately perform a 400-yard run (not necessarily a sprint). Grab water and rest 30 seconds before moving on to another exercise. The intensity is what matters—it is higher and more intense than interval training, and does not need to be timed.

Suggested Exercise Output

Children and Adolescents 6-17 Years:

Children and adolescents should do 60 minutes (1 hour) or more of physical activity daily.

 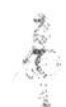

1. Aerobic: Most of the 60 or more minutes a day should be either moderate or vigorous aerobic activity, and should include vigorous activity at least 3 days a week.
2. Muscle-strengthening: As part of their 60 or more minutes of daily physical activity, children and adolescents should include muscle-strengthening physical activity on at least 3 days of the week.
3. Bone-strengthening: As part of their 60 or more minutes of daily physical activity, children and adolescents should include bone-strengthening physical activity on at least 3 days of the week.

Adults 18-64 Years:

For substantial health benefits, adults should do at least 150 minutes (2 hours and 30 minutes) a week of moderate-intensity activity.

a. 75 minutes (1 hour and 15 minutes) a week of vigorous-intensity aerobic physical activity, or an equivalent combination of moderate- and vigorous-intensity aerobic activity.
b. Aerobic activity should be performed in episodes of at least 10 minutes, and preferably, it should be spread throughout the week.
c. For more extensive benefits, adults should perform 300 minutes (5 hours) a week of moderate-intensity aerobic activity, 150 minutes a week of vigorous-intensity aerobic physical activity, or an equivalent combination of moderate- and vigorous-intensity activity.

Adults Over 65:

Older adults should perform activities that aid in prevention from falls and exercise according to their fitness level and quality of living.

Information provided by the FDA, 2016.

STEP 3: CHOOSE YOUR LEVEL OF FITNESS

Losing extra body fat takes time, hard work, and patience. No magic wand exists that will sprinkle fairy dust to make you lose 70 pounds at the end of these weeks together. Turning to impressive surgeries and pills can mask battles lurking deep within habits. The hard work of getting it off the right way and battling those root issues is sustainable, safe, and life-altering.

Choose which level you want to start with. On the following pages, you will find training programs for each level listed below.

Level 1	Level 2	Level 3
Beginner	**Intermediate**	**Advanced**
Injured or Recovering Needs modifications Taking it slower Older than 65 years	No/limited injuries Getting good at this Some modifications needed	Ready for anything Can hold plank 1 minute easy Comfortable around a gym

Below, you will see the different combinations of plans you can choose. Mix and match or try them a la carte.

Level List

Stretching	Level	**Walking**	Level
Stretcher Prepper Plan	1, 2, 3	Just Counting Steps	1
		Building Strength	1, 2, 3
Upper Body Plans		**Lower Body Plans**	
Upper Body Plus	2, 3	Bottoms Up Circuit 1	1, 2, 3
Upper Body Super Sets	2, 3	Bottoms Up Circuit 2	1, 2, 3
Upper Body Push	2, 3	Bottoms Up Circuit 3	1, 2, 3
Upper Body Pull	2, 3	Undie 500	2, 3
Core Only Plans		**Cardio Plans**	
Musical Core	1, 2, 3	You Choose Cardio	1, 2, 3
Core Circuits		Simply Moving	1, 2, 3
Core 1	1, 2, 3	Increase Cardio & Speed	1, 2, 3
Core 2	2, 3	Burst Training	1, 2, 3
Hard Core	3	Ninja Cardio Circuit	3
Scorpion Sting	3		
Total Body Plans		**Lower Body & Core Focused Plans**	
Boot Camp Circuit	1, 2, 3	Take A Chance	1, 2, 3
Countdown	2, 3	Butts & Guts	2, 3
HIT Countdown	3	Double Trouble	2, 3
Down & Back	3	4 Minute Rounds	2, 3

LEVEL 1 PROGRAM OPTION

Trainer Talk

Before you perform any exercise routine, warm up your body for a few minutes by walking or taking a few deep, full, slow breaths. Remember to progress at your own pace. If you are not ready to move forward to the suggested week, hang out at your current exercise routine and just repeat.

Level 1: Beginner 12 Week Exercise Program	**3 or up to 5 day plan**
Weeks 1 - 2 Stretcher Prepper Plan Just counting Steps	 M/W/F T/TH or M/W/F
Week 3 Stretcher Prepper Plan Building Strength	 T/TH M/W/F or T/TH
Week 4: Only move to the following week if your body is ready to do so. Otherwise, stay and progress at your own pace. Stretcher Prepper Plan Simply Moving	 M/W/F T/TH or M/W/F
Weeks 5 - 8 Stretcher Prepper Plan Increase Cardio & Seed or Bottoms Up Circuit 1	 T/TH M/W/F or T/TH
Weeks 9 - 12 Stretcher Prepper Plan You Choose Cardio or Bottoms Up Circuit 1 or Take A Chance Level 1	 T/TH M/W/F or T/TH

If you can only perform 3 days of exercise, you have the option to double up your exercise on those 3 days to maximize your workouts. If you have 5 days to exercise, you can break up your program as indicated above.

LEVEL 2 PROGRAM OPTION

Trainer Talk

Before you perform any exercise routine, warm up your body for a few minutes with one of the following: walk, front leg kicks, jumping jacks, jump rope.

Level 2: Intermediate 12 Week Full Body Program	**3 or up to 5 day plan**
Week 1	
Choose a Core Only Plan, Upper Body Plus or Pull, and the Stretcher Prepper Plan	M/W/F
Choose a Cardio Plan	T/TH or M/W/F
Weeks 2 - 3	
Choose a Lower Body Plan, a Core Only Plan, and Upper Body Plus or Sets	M/W/F
Choose a Cardio Plan	T/TH or M/W/F
Weeks 4-6	
Cardio Plan and Upper Body Plus or Sets	M/W/F
Lower Body Plan and Core Only Plan	T/TH or M/W/F
Weeks 7-9	
Choose a Total Body Plan and Upper Body Push/Pull	T/TH or M/W/F
Stretcher Prepper Plan and a Core Only Plan	M/W/F
Weeks 10-12	
Total Body Plan	M/W/F
Cardio Plan and a Core Only Plan	T/TH or M/W/F
Upper Body Push/Pull	T/TH or M/W/F

If you can only perform 3 days of exercise, you have the option to double up your exercise on those 3 days to maximize your workouts. If you have 5 days to exercise, you can break up your program as indicated above.

 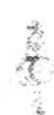

LEVEL 3 PROGRAM OPTION

Trainer Talk

Before you perform any exercise routine, warm up your body for a few minutes with one of the following: walk, front leg kicks, jumping jacks, jump rope.

Level 3: Advanced 12 Week Full Body Program 3 to 6 day plan

Week 1-6: Choose which exercise plan for each area you'd like to perform from the Level List. This makes it fresh so you can change up your workout often within these first 6 weeks.	
Choose any Upper Body Plan, a Lower Body Plan, and a Core Only Plan * Increase weight every 2 weeks	**M/W/F**
Choose any Cardio Plan and the Stretcher Prepper Plan	**T/TH**
You can combine the M/W/F and the T/TH/S plans on same day 3 times per week if time doesn't permit 6 days per week.	

Weeks 7-12: Continue with this program, choosing plans from the Level List.	
Choose one of the Lower Body & Core Focused Plans	**M/W/F**
Choose any Cardio Plan and an Upper Body Plan * Increase weight every 2 weeks	**T/TH/S**
You can combine the M/W/F and the T/TH/S plans on same day 3 times per week if time doesn't permit 6 days per week.	

If you can only perform 3 days of exercise, you have the option to double up your exercise on those 3 days to maximize your workouts. If you have 5 days to exercise, you can break up your program as indicated.

EXERCISE PLANS

All exercises marked with an asterisk (*) have a photo in the Program Exercise Descriptions section.

4 MINUTE ROUNDS

Perform each round with 1 minute per exercise with little to no rest between each exercise. Set up as fast as possible to start the next 4 minute round.

Round 1	**Round 6**
Slow Crunches	Flutter Crunches
Mountain Climbers	Flutter Squats
Lunge Pulses — Left	Lateral Walking Squats with Bands
Lunge Pulses — Right	Swimmers
Round 2	**Round 7**
Fast Crunches	Plank
Lateral Shuffle Hop	Star Jumps
Bridge Raises	All 4's Bent — Left
Bridge Inner Thighs Together	All 4's Bent — Right
Round 3	**Round 8**
L-Crunch — Left	Twisters
L-Crunch — Right	Sumo Side Kicks
180 Squat Twist	All 4's Straight Leg — Left
Dead Lifts	All 4's Straight Leg — Right
Round 4	**Round 9**
Surfers	Plank Middle Hip Dips
Jump Rope	Hot Potatoes — Left
Inner Thigh Lifts — Left	Hot Potatoes — Right
Inner Thigh Lifts — Right	Dead Lifts/Single Leg - Right/Left
Round 5	**Round 10**
Chuck 'N Tuck	Butt Squeezers
Squats with Weights	Pushups
Plie Squats	All 4's L-Lift — Right
Skaters	All 4's L-Lift — Left

Equipment Needed: Mat, medium hand weights, circle band, stability ball

BOOT CAMP

Perform each exercise for 1 minute. Catch your breath as you set up the next circuit and then dive right in. Level 1 can perform each exercise for 30 seconds.

Circuit 1

Bear Crawl
Burpees
Jogging Rear Kickers — forward & backward
Football Run

Circuit 2

Crab Walk — backward
High Knee Joggers — forward & backward
Skipping — as high as you can vertically
Mountain Climbers *

Circuit 3

Roman Walks
Surfers *
Lateral Shuffle Hop - back and forth
Plank *

Circuit 4

Jump Rope
Jumping Jacks
Plank High Fives*
Push Ups

Circuit 5

Squat Thrusts
Tricep Dips — on the floor or bench
Tuck Jumps or Jump Rope
Pogos *

Equipment Needed: Possible mat and jump rope.

BOTTOMS UP CIRCUITS

Perform 1,2 or all 3 of the circuits back to back. Rest as needed. If an exercise is single leg, perform second leg immediately after.

Weeks 1-6: 3 sets of 15	Weeks 7-12: 2 sets of 20

Circuit 1 - Perform 3 sets of 15 or 20

Deadlifts — both legs or single leg, left and right

Walking Lunges — optional stationary backward lunges, left and right

Sumo Side Kicks — left and right leg

Lateral Walking Squats with bands

All 4's L-Lifts — left and right leg *

Circuit 2 - Perform 3 sets of 15 or 20

Single Leg Reverse Lunges on Bench — left and right leg

Inner Thigh Lifts — flexed left and pointed left, repeat on right leg

Butt Squeezers — bands optional

All 4's Crossovers — left and right leg *

All 4's Straight Leg Lifts — left and right leg *

Circuit 3 - Perform 3 sets of 15 or 20

Bench Step Ups — add a kick at the top, left and right leg

Bench Side Step Ups — left and right leg

All 4's Bent Leg — left and right leg *

Plate Sliders Lunging Backwards — left and right leg

Plate Sliders Lunging Sideways — left and right leg

Equipment Needed: mat, weights, circle band, bench/step, paper plate, or furniture slider.

See exercise descriptions for modifications.

Building Strength

This is a perfect plan for those who might experience pain while walking longer bouts, or get stiff after walking. This plan lasts between 30 and 60 minutes depending on your walking time. It can be performed outside or on a cardio machine.

1	Walk at a warm up pace for 5 minutes.
2	Stop and perform standing stretch for 2 minutes. Stretch your major muscles, but don't lean over. Keep your head and heart above your hips.
3	Continue walking, but pick up the pace to a nice moderate brisk walk for 10-35 minutes.
4	Stop and perform standing stretch for 2 minutes. Stretch your major muscles, but keep your head and heart above your hips.
5	Continue brisk walking for 5-10 minutes.
6	Stop and perform 10 squats or backward lunges on each leg. Hold a handrail for support.
7	Continue walking, but slow to a cool down pace.
8	Stop and stretch for 3-5 minutes, focus on your lower back and legs, but especially the back of your legs (hamstrings).

Level 2 or 3 can perform this plan by jogging or running instead of walking.

Burst Training Levels 1, 2 or 3

Choose your level, then choose one of the three circuits in that level. Perform each exercise for one minute in that circuit with two minutes of rest between each.

Your goal is to get your heartrate as high as you should and as low as you can (recovering during the TWO full minutes of rest).

**Please note, this program is not for those who take medication for heart or blood pressure, or who are pregnant, have a metabolic disease, or are over 65 years of age. Please consult your physician if you have questions on if this type of exercise intensity is right for you.*

Choose Your Level

Level 1	
1	Skaters*, Stationary Backward Lunges, Front Kicks
2	Walking Stairs, Jogging, Jumping Jacks
3	Flutter Squat Taps*, Squats, Switch Squat Taps *
Level 2	
1	Prisoner Squat Kicks*, Prisoner Squats*, Skaters, Pogos*
2	Jumping Jacks, Football Runs in Place, Front Kicks, Mountain Climbers*
3	Football Run, Jogging Rear Kickers, Sumo Side Kicks, Jump Rope
Level 3	
1	Tuck Jumps, Skaters, High Knees, Burpees, Plank Hoppers*
2	Squat Thrusts, Pushups, Lunge Kicks, Plank Hoppers*, Star Jumps*
3	Prisoner Jumps*, Prisoner Squat Kicks, Pogos*, Burpees, Lateral Shuffle Hop

No equimpent needed.

Butts & Guts	
At the start of each circuit, begin a continuous clock. Perform each exercise for 20 seconds with only 10 seconds of rest before beignning the next exercise. Perform 2 rounds of the four exercises, then set up the next circuit and repeat the sequence with as little rest as possible.	
Cardio Circuit (repeat 1 time)	
1	Star Jumps*
2	Prisoner Squat Jumps*
3	Flutter Squats*
4	Skaters*
Legs Circuit (repeat 1 time)	
1	Pulse Lunges with 1 Kick — Left Leg
2	Pulse Lunges with 1 Kick — Right Leg
3	Jump Squats & 2 Stationary Squats
4	Lateral Shuffle Hop, immediatley repeat other direction*
Guts Circuit (repeat 1 time)	
1	Plank Left Side Dips (or hold for 20 seconds)
2	Plank Right Side Dips (or hold for 20 seconds)
3	Plank Middle Hip Dips*
4	Push Ups
Butts Circuit (right leg first round, left leg second round)	
1	All 4's Bent Leg *
2	All 4's Straight Leg*
3	All 4's L-Lift*
4	All 4's Crossover*

Equipment Needed: mat. See exercise descriptions for modifications.

CORE CIRCUITS

Perform one set and go to the next exercise, then repeat the circuit as indicated.

CORE 1	
10 x 2	Bent Leg Raises*
10 x 2	Surfers*
10 x 2	Twisters*
10 x 2	Plank Middle Plank Hip Dips*
10 x 2	YTWL*
CORE 2	
20 x 2	Band (or Ball) Pass Off
20 x 2	Seal Crunches*
20 x 2	Chuck 'N Tuck*
20 x 2	Bicycles
20 x 2	Butt Squeezers
HARD CORE	
50 x 1	Flutters Crunches*
50 x 1	Side Plank Thread the Needle — Left
50 x 1	Side Plank Thread the Needle — Right
50 x 1	Swimmers
50 x 1	Star Crunches

Equipment Needed: mat, stability ball. See exercise descriptions for modifications.

COUNTDOWN

Perform number (on left) of exercises (on right).

100	Jumping Jacks — as fast as possible
90	Squats
80	Rainbows - 40 each leg
70	Crunches*
60	Step Ups on Bench - 30 each leg
50	Push Ups*
40	Tricep Dips
30	Donkey Kicks* or Handstand Kick Ups*
20	Plank Knee to Elbow — 20 each side
10	Burpees

Equipment Needed: mat, optional weight, bench or step. See exercise descriptions for modifications.

DOUBLE TROUBLE

Perform 20 of everything, and then do it again! If left and right leg, perform 20 on each. Level 1: Only perform 20 of each exercise.

Option 1: Go through Bottom Circuit and repeat before going to Core.

Option 2: Go through Bottom Circuit and Core Circuit, then repeat.

WARM UP

Jumping jacks, front kicks, jog in place, or take a few flights of stairs for a few minutes.

BOTTOM: Need a deadlift weight, circle band, stability ball, and mat

1 Pogos Left & Right Legs*
2 Switch Squats*
3 Walking Lunges (or Stationary Backward Lunges)
4 Flutter Squats*
5 Lateral Walking Squats with Bands
6 Deadlifts
7 Bottoms Up on Stability Ball*
8 Hamstring Bridge on the Stability Ball — laying on floor, feet on ball*
9 All 4's L-Lift Right & Left*
10 All 4's Bent Leg — Right & Left*
11 All 4's Straight Leg — Right & Left*
12 All 4's Crossed Leg — Right & Left*

CORE: Need a stability ball, small core weight, circle band, mat

1 Chuck 'N Tuck*
2 Reverse Crunch
3 Plank on Stability Ball — hold for 20 seconds*
4 Butt Squeezers — bands are optional
5 Oblique Lifts*
6 Twisters*
7 Side Plank — hold for 20 seconds on each side
8 Swimmers — go slow

Equiment Needed: mat, hand weights, circle band, stability ball

DOWN & BACK

Perform number (on left) of exercises (on right).

60	Jumping Jacks — as fast as possible
50	Plie Squats — weighted if possible*
40	Side Lunges — 20 on each leg
30	Plank Tappers*
20	Step Ups on Bench - 20 on each leg
10	Star Jumps*
20	Prisoner Jumps*
30	Pogos — 15 on each leg*
40	Lunges — 20 of each leg
50	Push Ups*
60	Butt Kickers

Equipment Needed: mat

Trainer Talk:

This is a quick 30 minute or less cardio workout that compliments an upper body program.

HIIT COUNTDOWN

Perform number (on left) of exercises (on right).

100	Step Ups on Bench — 50 each leg
90	Crunches*
80	Butt Kickers — 80 each leg
70	Plank Knee to Elbow — 70 each leg
60	High Knee Joggers - 60 each leg
50	Butt Squeezers
40	Plank Middle Hip Dips — 40 each side*
30	Skaters — 30 each side*
20	Pogos — 20 each leg*
10	Decline Pushups

Equipment Needed: mat

Increase Your Cardio Output & Speed

Use any cardio machine or do outside cardio. Increase your incline or speed for four weeks.

Warm Up - easy effort	**5 minutes**
Moderate Effort (incline or speed)	**5 minutes**
Recovery (lower incline or speed or both)	**1 minutes**
Hard Effort (Speed)	**3 minutes**
Moderate Effort (decline from speed)	**5 minutes**
Hard Effort (Speed)	**3 minutes**
Recovery	**1 minutes**
Moderate Effort (incline or speed)	**5 minutes**
Cool Down	**2 minutes**
Stretch Major Muscles	**5 minutes**

Just Counting Steps

This plan is for those who are brand new to fitness, have an injury, are 65 years old or older, or have to go very slow for any reason. It can help get muscles moving and build endurance for other activities in the future. Generally speaking, just counting steps throughout the day will not help people lose a lot of body fat. Talk to your doctor about what is right for you personally, but here are some general guidelines.

1. 2,000 steps is roughly 1 mile, depending on your stride.

If you have access to a high school track, you can count how many steps it takes you to walk one lap. Multiply this by four and you'll have an estimated mile step count - as long as you keep those strides up for all four laps.

2. An average goal is 10,000 total steps per day.

Your daily step goal will be different than others. 10,000 is an estimated daily goal of total steps, not just including exercise steps. Setting an everyday step goal can help many with heart-healthy goals.

3. Track your progress.

See if you can go longer with distance or time as you gain stamina and strength. If you find you are sore or tired from pushing yourself the day prior, take it easy and allow your body to rest so you can go after your goal the following day.

Musical Core

Your goal is to listen to music and just feel the beat by performing the core exercises for a minimum of 2 counts of 8. Make it a goal to hit 4 counts of 8!

1	Fast Crunches
2	Reverse Crunches
3	Fast Crunches
4	Bicycles
5	Fast Crunches
6	Swimmers
7	Fast Crunches
8	Plank Middle Hip Dips*
9	Fast Crunches
10	L-Crunch — Left
11	Fast Crunches
12	L-Crunch — Right
13	Fast Crunches

Equipment Needed: mat

Ninja Cardio Circuit

Perform the exercise on left for a few seconds and switch to the one on the right for a few seconds. Go back and forth for a total of one minute. Then go to the next exercise with only one minute of rest Once finished with the four minute circuit, rest one minute and repeat one or two more times. Level 2 perform 30 seconds of each.

Warm up major muscles for a few minutes.

1	1 min. on	2 Prisoner Jumps*	1 Star Jump*	1 min. rest
2	1 min. on	1 Handstand*	1 Pushup*	1 min. rest
3	1 min. on	2 Donkey Kick Claps*	2 Mountain Climbers*	1 min. rest
4	1 min. on	2 Squat Thrusts	2 Flutter Squats*	1 min. rest

Rest and repeat up to 2 more times.

Equipment Needed: mat

Scorpion Sting

4 sets (one on each side) of scorpions followed by 1 minute of the next exercise.

4 sets	**Scorpions***
1 minute	**Plank Left Side**
4 sets	**Scorpions**
1 minute	**Plank Middle**
4 sets	**Scorpions**
1 minute	**Plank Right Side**
4 sets	**Scorpions**
1 minute	**Plank Middle Hip Dips***
4 sets	**Scorpions**
1 minute	**Plank Left Side Dips**
4 sets	**Scorpions**
1 minute	**Plank Right Side Dips**
4 sets	**Scorpions**

Equipment Needed: mat

Simply Moving

Increase your incline or speed weekly for 4 weeks.

Preferably on a track or outside on the sidewalk. Any cardio machine will do.		
Warm Up	Easy	5 minutes
Speed Walk	Moderate	1 minute
Jog	Moderate — Hard	3 minutes
Run	Hard Effort (Speed)	5 minutes
Jog	Moderate — Hard	3 minutes
Speed Walk	Moderate	1 minute
Cool Down	Easy	5 minutes

STRETCHER PREPPER PLAN

STRETCHER PREPPER PLAN flows from one exercise to the next. Make a goal for your daily stretching - first thing in the morning, after lunch, or before bed. Choose all or some stretches that feel good to your body. Avoid anything that lends weird tingles, twinges, or agitations.

Stretches

Hold each exercise 15 - 45 seconds or 5-6 full breaths.

1	**Full Body Stretch***
2	**Knees To Chest ***
3	**One Knee To Chest ***
4	**Hamstring Stretch***
5	**L-Stretch***
6	**Drop to Side***
7	**Glute Stretch ***
8	**Round & Arch Back***
9	**Child's Sit***
10	**Back Extension***
11	**Reverse Bridge***
12	**Forward Fold***
13	**Standing Inhale Stretch**

Equipment Needed: mat

0

Take A Chance	
Level 1: Roll 2 dice and perform the corresponding exercises. Perform 1-2 of each number. Levels 2 & 3: Roll 2 dice and perform the corresponding exercises. Once you hit 3 of the same number, cross it off the list.	
2	2 sets of 24 each: Inner Thigh Lifts flexed foot & pointed foot
3	3 rounds of 3: Star Jumps*, Pulse Squats, Pushups
4	4 rounds of 4: Lunge Kick Backs, Curtsey Lunges, Curtsey Kicks
5	5 rounds of 8: Plie Squats Right Heel Up, Plie Left Heel Up, Plie Both Heels Up*
6	2 rounds of 8 sets: Lateral Walking Squats L/R and Standing Band Leg Raises L/R
7	8 R/L: Pogos L, Pogos R*, Mountain Climbers*, Knee to Elbow
8	1 round L, 1 round R 16: Lying Leg Lifts, Rainbows*, Potatoes, Clams
9	16 R/L: L-Crunches, Crunches, Reverse Crunches
10	16 All 4's: Bent Leg, Straight Leg, Crossover, L-Lifts*
11	16 Side Plank Dips L/M/R
12	12 sets: 1 Burpee into 2 Plank Tappers*

M = Middle, L = Left side, R = Right side, L/R = Left and then right side

Equipment Needed: mat, circle band

Undie 500

Perform the 3 circuits back to back. Drink water and rest as needed.

Circuit #1 - 150 Exercises		
50	Lunge Kick Ups	25 each leg — lunge back & kick
25	Pogos*	13 on each leg
25	Star Jumps*	Oh baby — enjoy!
50	Prisoner Squat Kicks*	25 each leg
Circuit #2 - 150 Exercises		
50	On The Beach*	Oblique crunch — 25 laying on each side
50	L-Crunches	50 each leg — pace yourself!
25	Butt Squeezers	Use band if possible on ankles
25	Bridge Raises	Keep knees together for another 25 for an extra burn
Circuit #3 - 200 Exercises		
50	Lateral Walking Squats with Bands	50 each way — SQUAT LOW, bands on ankles
50	All 4's Bent Leg*	50 on each leg — try different styles too
50	Inner Thigh Lifts	50 each leg — bands optional with point & flex
50	Curtsey Lunge	50 of each leg — kick or tap for extra fun

Equipment Needed: mat, circle band

Upper Body Plans

Weeks 1-6 Option 1: Perform 12 of each exercise, then move to the next exercise. After all five exercises, repeat to the top and perform 10 of each. Repeat with 8.

Upper Body Plus: Perform 3 sets of 12, 10, 8	
1	Back: Bent-over Rows
2	Chest: Pushups & Flyes
3	Shoulders: Overhead Press & Upright Rows
4	Biceps: Curls & Hammer
5	Triceps: Pulldowns & Extensions

Weeks 1-6 Option 2: Perform each circuit 3 times, then move to the next circuit. Level 1 perform only the first set of 10 for the first 2 weeks, then add the rest.

Upper Body Super Sets: Perform each circuit 3 sets of 10	
Circuit 1	Pull Ups & Bent-over Rows
Circuit 2	Slow Biceps & Tricep Extensions
Circuit 3	Lateral Shoulder Raise & Front Shoulder Raise
Circuit 4	Pushups & Reverse Flyes

Weeks 7-12: Perform these two every other day. If you miss a day, still continue with the next plan that is orignially due on that day.

Upper Body Push: Increase your weight with less repetitions — 12, 10, 8, 6	
Tomorrow perform Upper Body Pull	
1	Shoulders: Lateral Raise or Reverse Flyes
2	Triceps: Kick Backs
3	Back: Bent-over Rows
4	Chest: Flye Crunches* or Pushups
5	Triceps: Tricep Dips or Extensions
Upper Body Pull: Increase your weight with less repetitions — 12, 10, 8, 6	
Tomorrow perform Upper Body Push	
1	Biceps: Hammer Curls or Bicep Curls
2	Back: Pull Ups or Lat Pull Downs - Machine
3	Upper Body: Seated Rows or Bent-over Rows

Equipment Needed: your hand weights will vary as you progress with your routine. Begin with light to moderate weights.

You Choose Cardio

Determine how long you have to physically perform cardio today. I suggest 30-60 minutes. Don't foget to choose cardio options that make you smile!

- Go outside for a run
- Get on a treadmill, elliptical, stairs, seated bike, or any other machine
- Play racquetball, tennis, pickelball
- Play ping pong
- Go geocaching or try some type of scavenger hunt and walk or jog to the places
- Go swimming, water skiing, tubing, knee boarding, or water sports
- Go body surfing, windsailing, wave catching
- Plug in a fitness DVD and perform the fitness class
- Go rock climbing or hiking
- Find a trampoline park or jump on your own
- Find a local fitness or group cycling class
- Take a bike ride somewhere new
- Put on those roller blades
- Find a pick up game of basketball or shoot hoops
- Grab your family and play old fashioned tag at the park
- Call a neighbor (or AP) and go for a brisk walk
- Take one of the cardio programs from this book

EXERCISE DESCRIPTIONS AND PHOTOS

Stretcher Prepper Program Descriptions

Exercises are listed specifically in sequential order.

1. *Full Body Stretch* – Lie flat on the floor on your back, arms raised above the head, which is touching the floor. Extend your body fully, like it is being pulled in opposite directions.

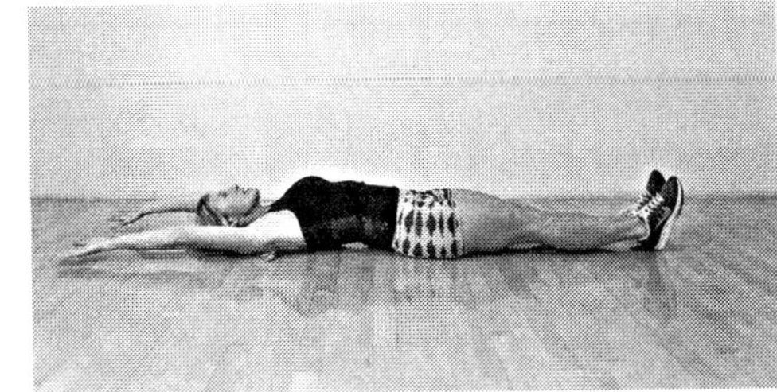

2. *Knees to Chest* – from the first exercise, continue through by bringing knees to chest, allowing your lower back to sink into the floor. *Lift your neck and shoulders and curl your chin to your chest for added benefit.

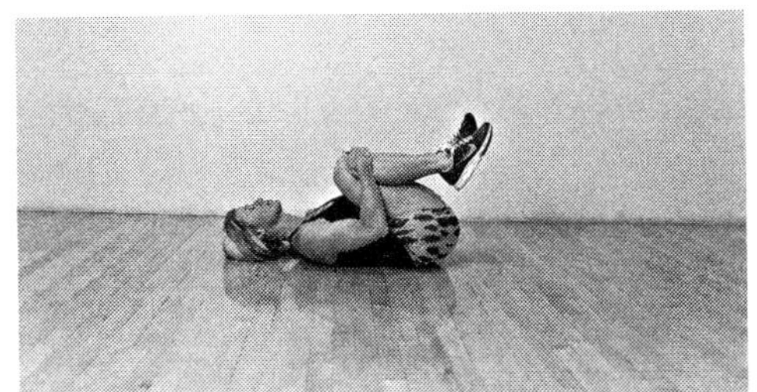

3. *One Knee to Chest* – from Knees to Chest position, drop only your left leg, so it rests and relaxes on the floor, like the first "Prone Stretch." Keep your right knee bent and pulled up to your chest. Gently grab your right knee with your left hand and pull your knee across your chest, leaving your shoulders comfortably close to the ground. Breathe slowly for 5-6 breaths. Transition to the other leg slowly and repeat the stretch on the other side. *Straighten the bent knee while pulled across your chest.

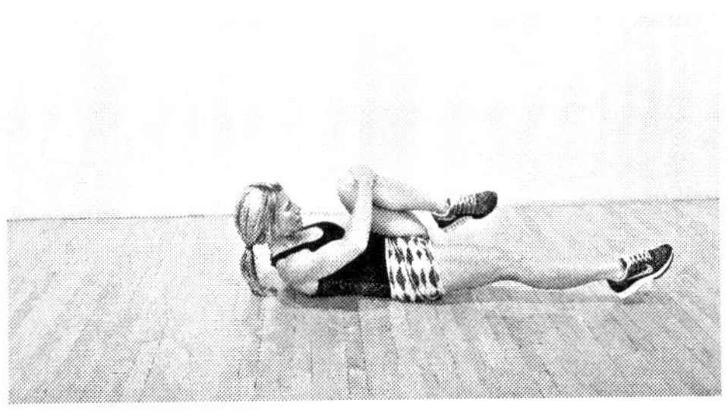

4. *Hamstring Stretch* – Lying on your back, slowly bring up your legs as close as you can to your chest, keeping them as straight as possible.

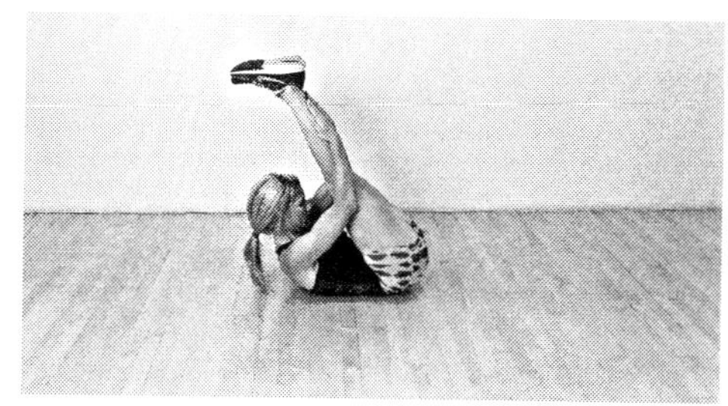

5. *L-Stretch* – while in the ending stretch position from the Hamstring Stretch, lie back down to the floor, but bend your knees and put your feet flat on the floor. Take one leg and drape it over the other to make an 'L.' Grab your bottom leg or bottom ankle if flexibility allows. Remain there for 5-6 breaths. Then switch sides. *Point and flex your toes while in the stretch for a deeper approach.

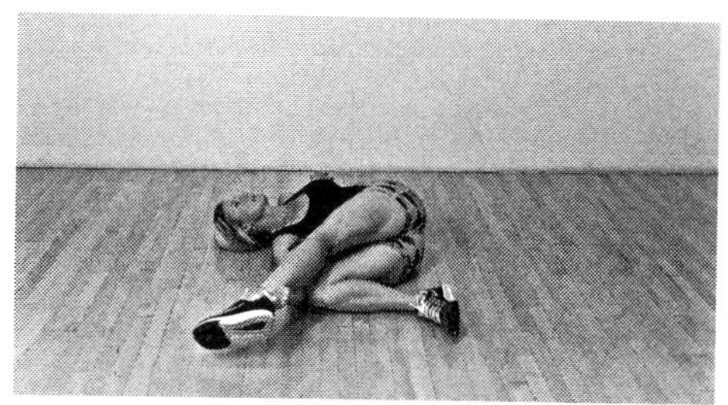

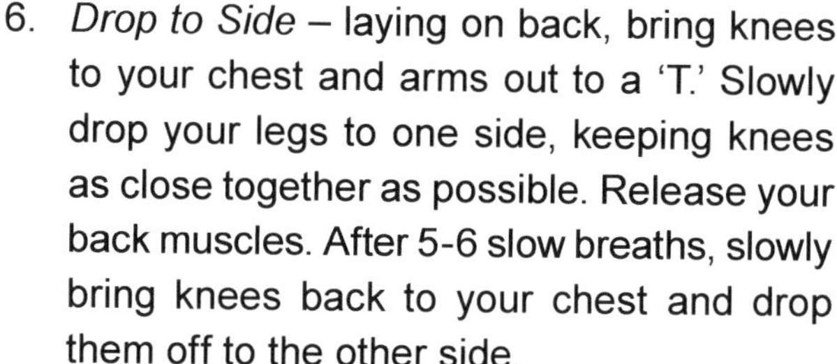

6. *Drop to Side* – laying on back, bring knees to your chest and arms out to a 'T.' Slowly drop your legs to one side, keeping knees as close together as possible. Release your back muscles. After 5-6 slow breaths, slowly bring knees back to your chest and drop them off to the other side.

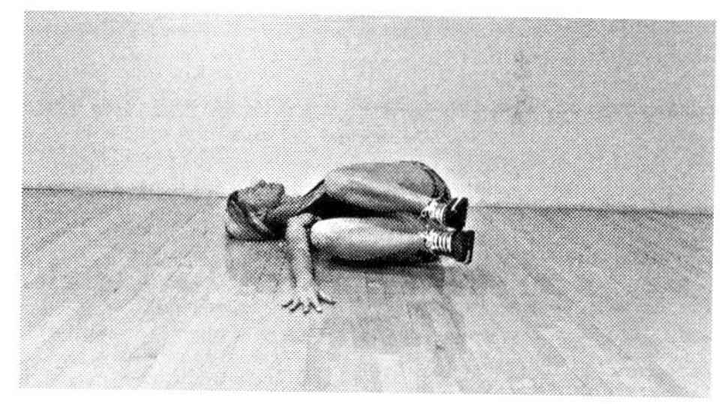

7. *Glute Stretch* – Lie back down on your back with knees bent and feet flat on the floor. Take your right leg and place the right ankle on the left knee. Using your hands, pull up on the bottom of your left thigh, so your left foot comes off the floor. Relax your muscles as you stretch. Breathe 5-6 full breaths before releasing the hands and exchanging to the other leg. *Extend the knee that has the ankle on it and grab your calf instead of your thigh.

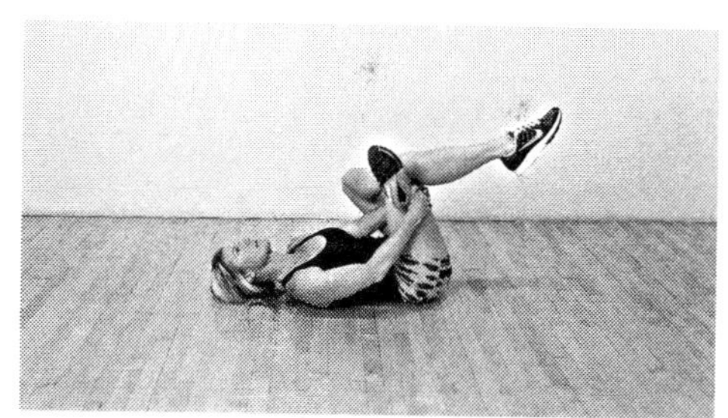

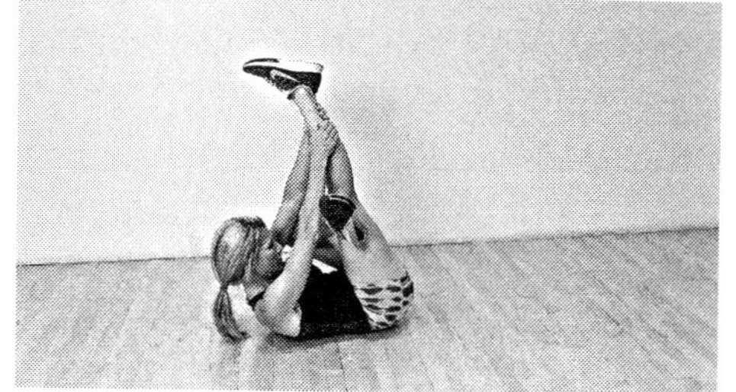

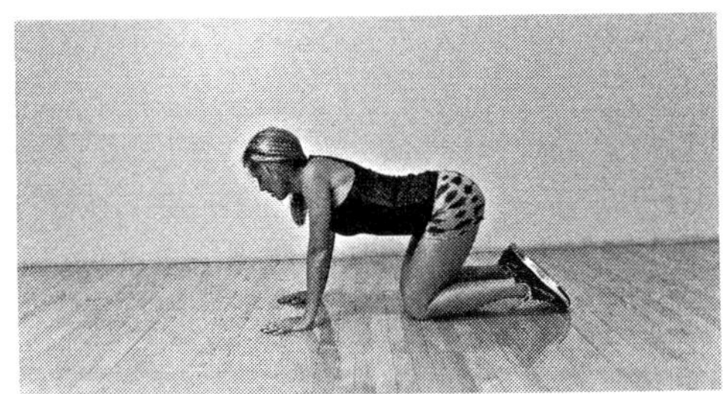

8. *Round and Arch Back* – transition to hands and knees on the floor. Keep hands aligned under your shoulders and your knees aligned under your hips. Slowly lower your chin towards your chest and round your back, exhaling all your air. Separate your shoulders as you press your spine toward the ceiling. Hold as long as you can before needing to inhale. As you inhale, relax your back and neck by slightly looking up and arching your back. Repeat these two motions as you breathe in and out, up to 6 times.

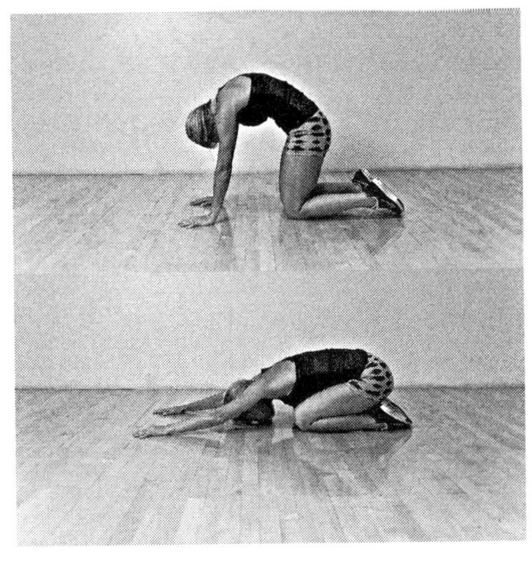

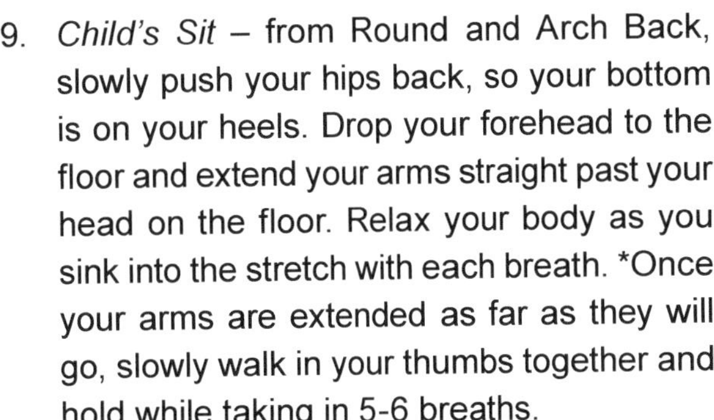

9. *Child's Sit* – from Round and Arch Back, slowly push your hips back, so your bottom is on your heels. Drop your forehead to the floor and extend your arms straight past your head on the floor. Relax your body as you sink into the stretch with each breath. *Once your arms are extended as far as they will go, slowly walk in your thumbs together and hold while taking in 5-6 breaths.

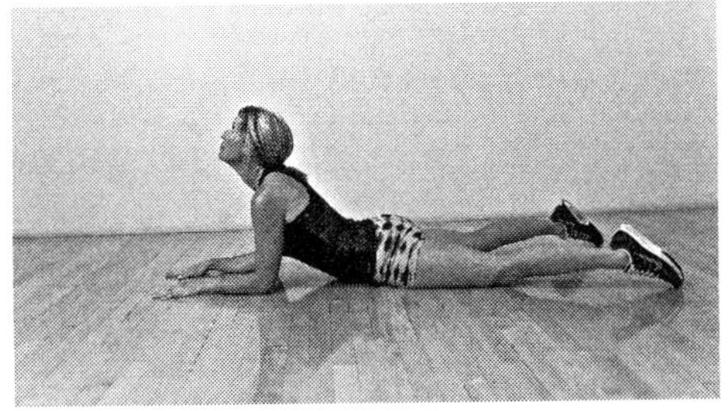

10. *Back Extension* – from Child's Sit, slowly push your hips forward into a plank-like position, but drop your hips to the ground. Arms should be under your shoulders with bent elbows. Look towards the ceiling as you breathe out and stretch your abdominal muscles and neck. Relax the bottom half of your body. Skip this stretch if it irritates your back.

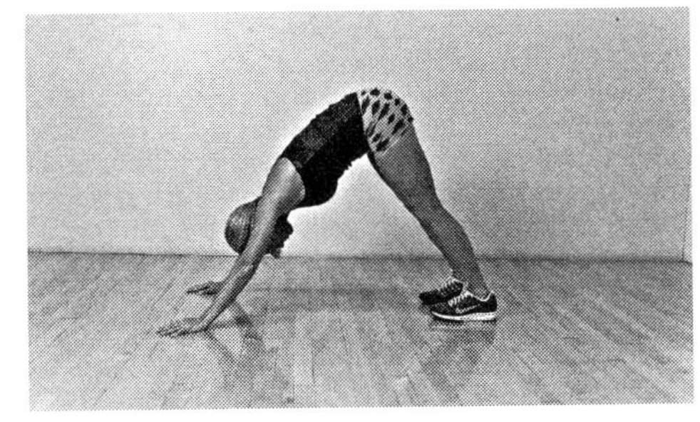

11. *Reverse Bridge* – from Back Extension, push your hips up in the air and slightly walk your hands closer to your feet as you place your weight evenly on your feet and hands. Relax your shoulders and neck and breathe slowly for 5-6 breaths. *Aim to place your heels flat on the ground while in this position.

12. *Forward Fold* – from Reverse Bridge, place weight on your feet by walking your hands toward your feet to a standing position (slightly bend your knees if the stretch is too deep). Keep your head down, face your eyes towards your legs and the crown of your head towards the ground. Pull upper body towards your legs and wrap your hands around your legs. Hold for 5-6 breaths, then very slowly round your back as you come to a standing position. *Aim to place your hands flat on the floor or tucked under your feet (palms up).

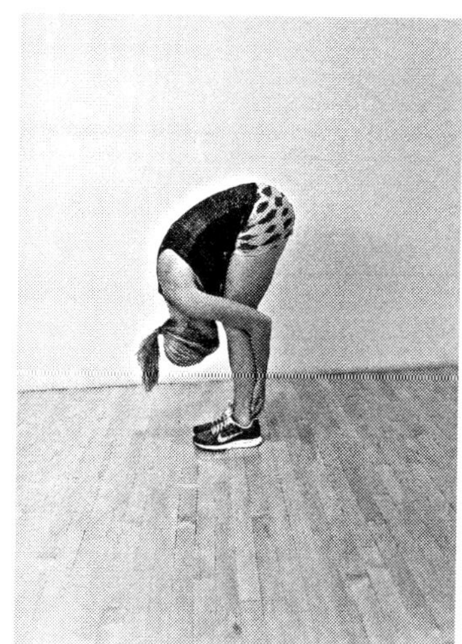

13. *Standing Inhale Stretch* – stand up tall with feet wider than shoulder width. Slowly exhale all air while you squat and scoop down with your arms to cross in front of your body, slightly brushing the floor without bending over if possible. Inhale as you stand up and reach arms all the way up overhead, opened wide, looking towards heaven—as high as you can reach. Repeat as soon as you need to exhale. Continue 5-6 times. *Aim for holding it at the top with full lungs as long as you can before exhaling and coming slowly back down.

Program Exercise Descriptions

Any time you perform exercises, do them deliberately, slowly, and controlled. Think about the actual muscles you are targeting and always breathe in and out—never hold your breath. Remember to always warm up your body before exercise, aim to drink about 3 ounces of water every 20 minutes, and always stretch when you are finished exercising.

1. *180 Squat Twists.* In a deep squat position, jump up in the air and turn 180 degrees before landing in a deep squat (180 degrees in the other direction). Use your arms to propel the motion. Keep your knees behind your toes. Repeat the same way you came so you do not become dizzy. This is a great cardio booster!

2. *All 4's Bent Leg:* Start on your hands and knees. Keep your head and neck neutral while looking at the floor. Engage your core and place one leg bent in the air. Flex your foot and press your heel towards the ceiling. Keep your back and arms straight. Repeat this as you focus the exercise on your rear end, hamstring, and slightly in your lower back. If you feel it more in your lower back, do not lift as high. Keep your hips facing the ground at all times.

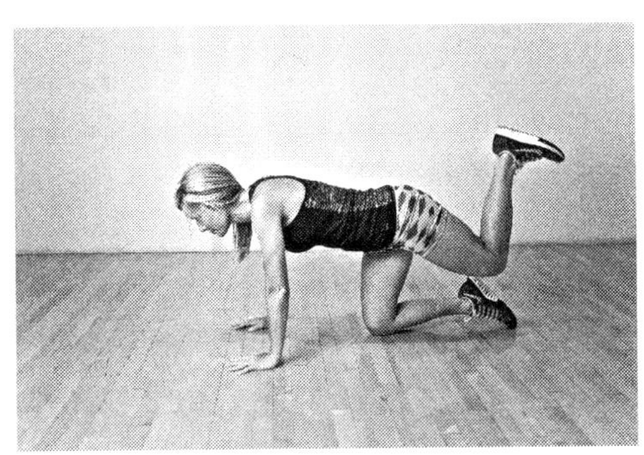

3. *All 4's L-Lift:* Same as All 4's Bent Knee except you will take your leg and turn it so your heel faces your rear end and your knee faces opposite your hip. It will look like an 'L' that you will lift up and down.

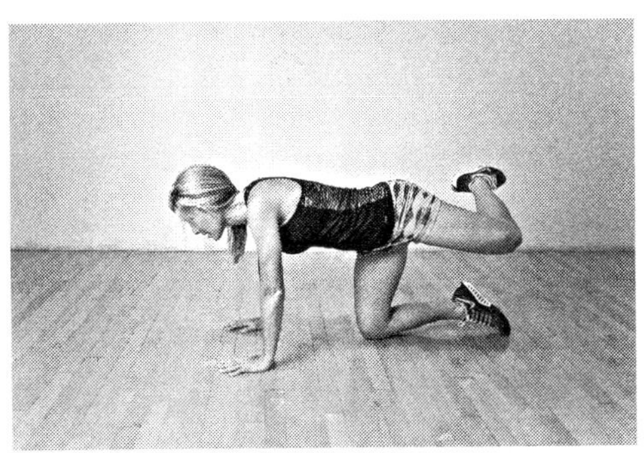

4. *All 4's Straight Leg:* Same as Bent Leg, but straighten your leg and flex your foot.

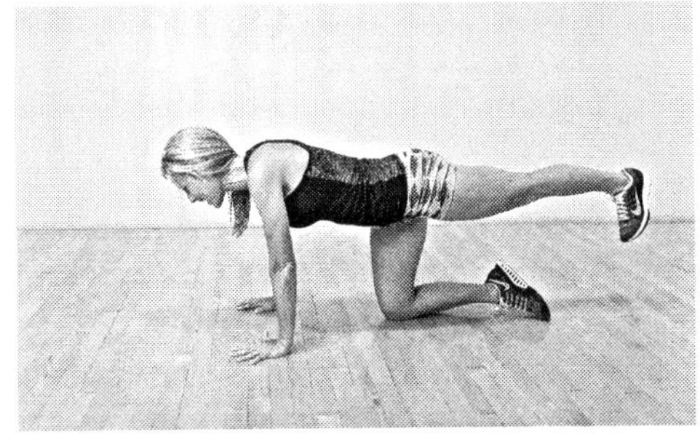

5. *All 4's Crossovers:* Start in All 4's Bent Knee position and cross your knee over the other knee and then back. You do not need to touch the floor with your knee. You should feel a good stretch in your hip.

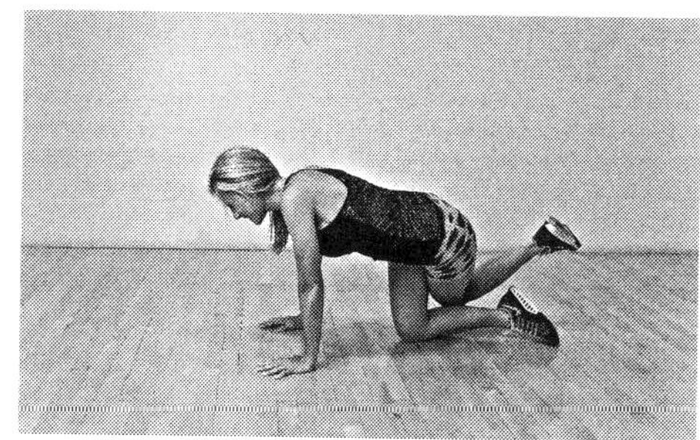

6. *Band (or Ball) Pass Off:* Lie on your back and hold a ball or exercise band. Reach your hands above your head and extend your entire body to a full stretch position. Crunch and pass the ball from your hands to your feet. Extend your entire body and then reverse the exercise and pass the ball back to your hands. Repeat.

7. *Bench Step Ups/Side Step Ups:* Use a bench, stool, or chair that is sturdy enough for your weight, step up with your left foot and then with the right, meeting the left foot on top. As you step up, press through the heel and keep your core braced. Standing together with both feet on the apparatus, reverse the exercise by taking the right leg to the ground first. Take the left leg down to the ground and then repeat this sequence. This will target the left leg muscles if you repeat on this same leg for a period of time before going to the right leg. *Bench Side Step Ups:* Same as Bench Step Ups, except you will step up from the side.

8. *Bent-over Rows:* Lean over and draw in your abs, keeping knees soft and bent. Exhale as you pull your arms in and up, squeezing elbows together towards your belly. As you drop your arms back down, keep your back flat. Do not drop your shoulders.

9. *Bicep Curl:* Alternate arms, slowly curl all the way up close to the shoulder and all the way down close to the thighs. Keep elbows touching your sides without moving them. **If you don't feel it in your biceps by rep 8, make sure your core is engaged and your elbows are not swinging, or choose a heavier weight.*

10. *Bicycles:* As shown in the first picture, keep one of your shoulder blades on the ground and rotate your shoulder and elbow towards your opposite knee. You have the option to extend one leg and suspend it off the ground or allow it to touch the ground. *Level 1 (Reclining):*

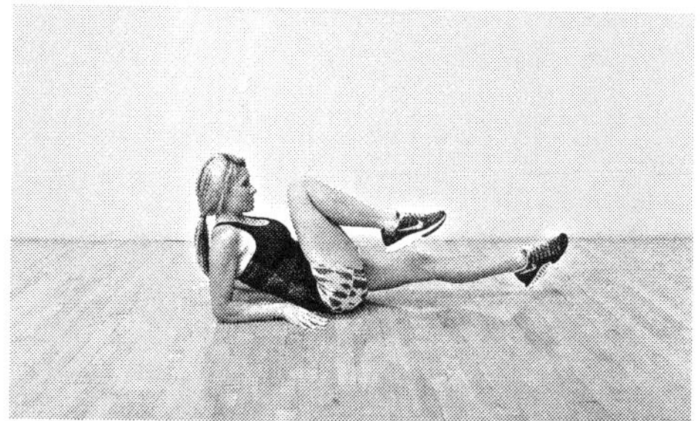

Lounge back, secure your body with your elbows, but chest high to keep from dropping. Bend left leg towards chest. Take the opposite leg, either suspended or on the ground, and switch legs as you exhale and inhale. You can go quick or slow with this one. *Level 3:* As shown in the third picture, keep your chest raised as you sit on your glutes instead of laying back. Rotate back and forth as you bring your knees to your chest.

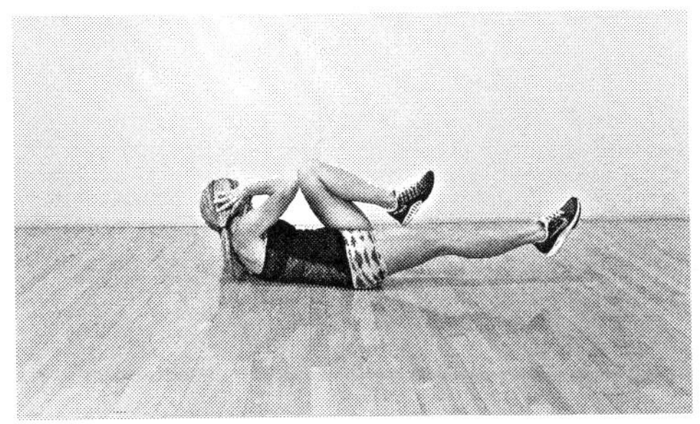

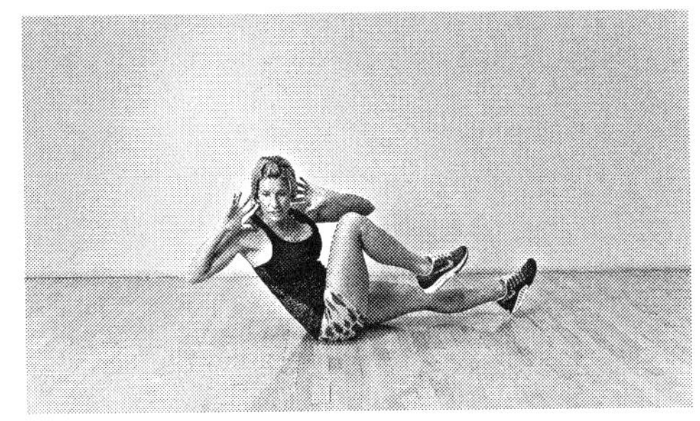

11. *Bottoms Up on Ball:* Use a large stability ball. Place your hips on the ball and your hands on the floor. Slightly turn in your heels so they point towards each other. Keep your legs hip distance apart. Slowly raise your lower half up in the air and squeeze your rear end. Slowly bring your legs down with the same speed you raised them. Resist gravity. You should feel this more in your legs than your lower back. If there is too much pressure in your lower back, do not lift as high.

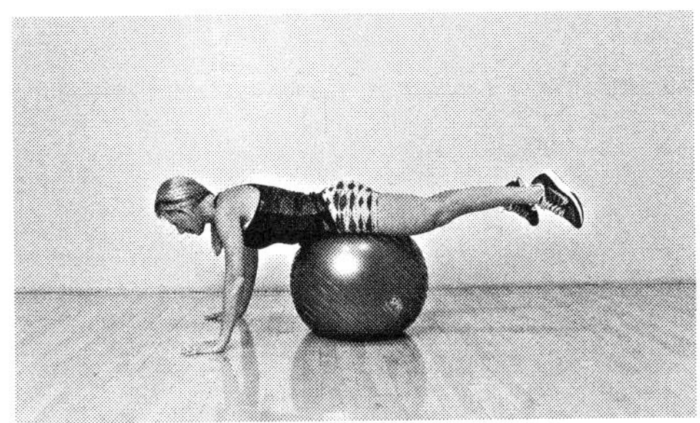

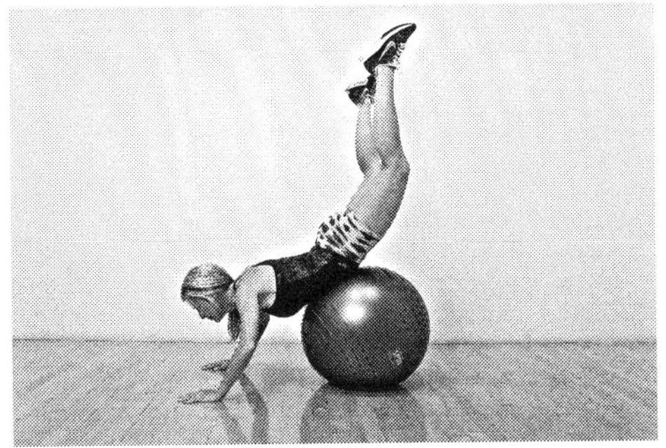

12. *Bridge Raises/Inner Thighs Together:* Lie on your back with your knees bent and feet flat on the floor. Keep your knees hip width apart. Raise your hips off the ground. Lift as high as you need to without putting too much pressure on your back. Then, lower your hips to the ground. *Inner Thighs Together:* For a harder intensity, keep your knees together while you lift and lower and lift your toes up off the ground.

13. *Burpees:* Stand upright, jump high in the air with hands overhead and as you land, squat and catch the floor with your hands and legs. Hop your legs out to a plank position. *Level 1:* Take the hop out and march the feet out to the plank position one at a time instead of the hop. *Level 3:* Add a quick pushup after you hit a plank, then bring feet back in and jump off the floor to repeat.

14. *Butt Squeezers:* Lie on your stomach and bend your arms. Lie your forehead on the back of your overlapped hands. Relax your upper body and lift your kneecaps off the ground while keeping your legs somewhat straight. Squeeze legs together and apart. Repeat this at a comfortable speed. Focus on your glutes, lower back, and hamstrings.

15. *Chuck 'N Tuck:* Lie on your back holding a stability ball. Chuck the ball in the air and catch it, using momentum. Holding the ball in front of you, lift your body upward to sit up while bringing your knees to your chest. Touch the balls to your feet and then unfold and lie back down, holding the ball to your chest. Repeat. *Level 1:* Stay on your back the entire exercise and only bring up your legs instead of your upper body. *Level 3:* Try to keep your head, shoulders, and legs off the ground throughout the entire exercise.

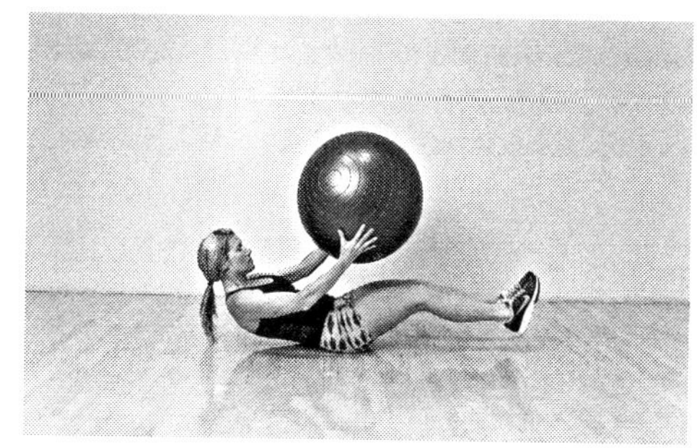

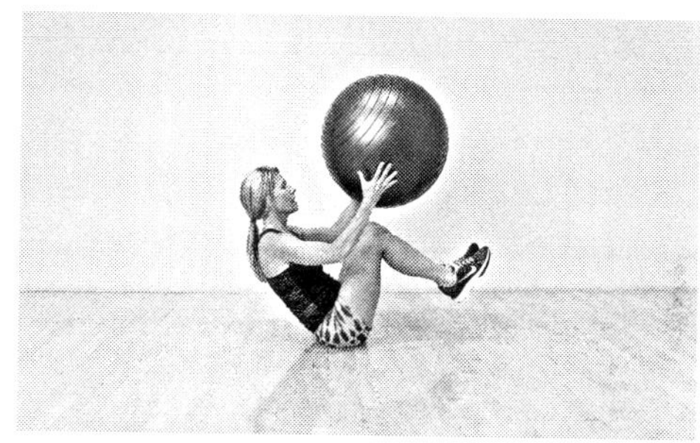

16. *Clams*: Lie on the ground on your side, keep both knees and ankles together. Dip your knees to the ground and lift your feet in the air. Slowly open your knees while keeping your bottom knee on the ground. Keep your feet in the air and do not disconnect your feet—keep them together at all times. Bring your knee back down to the starting position. Repeat. Make this harder by adding a circle band around your thighs.

17. *Crunches:* Lie on your back, knees bent and feet on the floor, slightly lift your head and tuck it as if you are holding an apple between your chin and chest. Keep eyes looking over your knees. Position hands behind your head, slightly cradling your head. Relax your neck. Breathe air out as you lift and inhale as you come back down. Lift your chest. Your head, shoulders, and arms should come along for the ride. Keep your lower back pressed in the ground. Legs can be down or up and bent hovering over your hips.

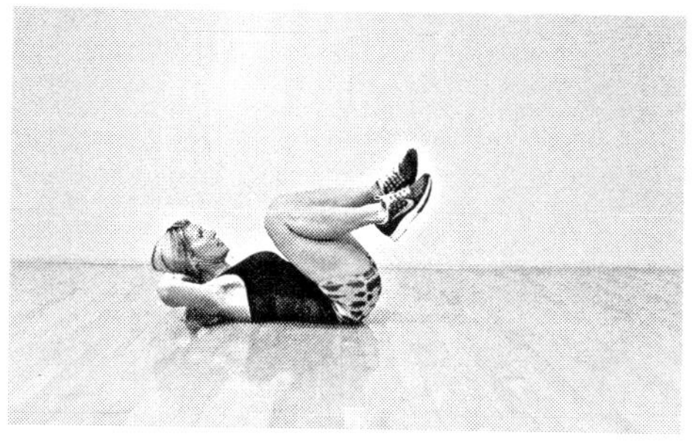

18. *Curtsey Lunges/Kicks:* Start in a right lunge. Adjust your back left leg so it stands crossed behind your other leg—like a curtsey bow. You can pulse or perform a single lunge in this position. If this irritates your knees, do not cross back as far. *Kicks:* After you reach back and curtsey, take your back left leg and kick it off to the left side and then go back to its starting position. Never straighten your legs all the way. It is a tricky balance move and very good for your legs and core.

19. *Deadlifts/Single Leg:* These are still a great fundamental exercise. Stand with feet slightly apart. Option to use weight. Hinge forward at the hips with a flat back and engaged core. Keep your neck neutral and have your eyes follow the movement. Keep your core engaged and braced. Slightly bend your knees for less pressure on your back. The lighter the weight, the straighter your legs can be. The heavier the weight, the more bend is required in the knees. This is a good exercise that targets your rear end, hamstrings, and lower back. *It is very important to note, this can strain your back if it is not performed correctly and with proper weight. For questions on this exercise, please see a local health professional. *Single Leg:* Perform the same exercise except only use one leg. If you keep your right leg on the ground, slightly bend it if needed, and take your other leg up off the ground as you bend at the hips. Repeat on the same leg for desired reps, then repeat on the opposite side.

20. *Donkey Kicks/Claps:* Squat with hands and feet on the floor, without knees actually touching the floor. Kick your legs up overhead (or as high/low as you feel comfortable). As soon as you land softly, repeat. The first time may be rough, but you will slowly get the hang of it. This is a huge cardio boost, so be ready. Repeat. *Level 1:* If you are not ready to take both legs up, lift one at a time and become used to how high your leg can go. If you are ready to jump a little, go for it. It does not have to be super high. *Level 3 (Claps):* After you land from your Donkey Kick, push back on your heels and lift your hands off the ground for a quick clap. Immediately repeat and perform another Donkey Kick.

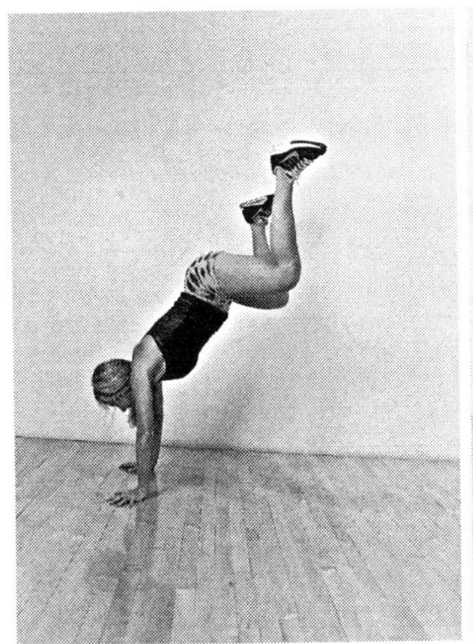
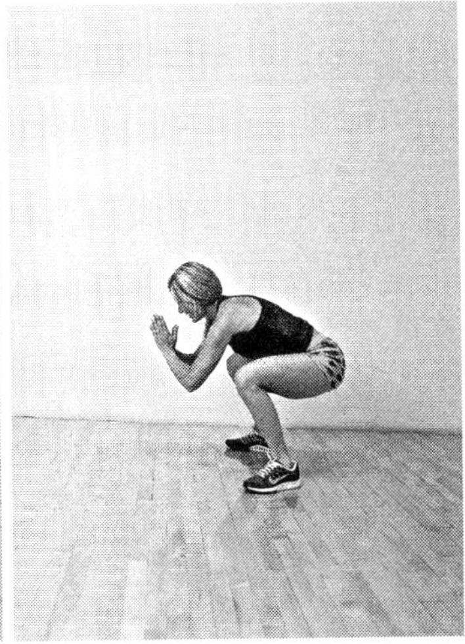
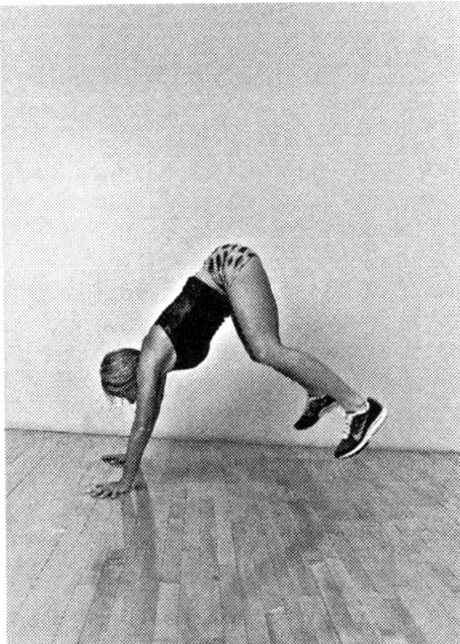

21. *Fast Crunches:* Same description as Crunches, but go faster with a little less range of motion.

22. *Flutter Crunches:* Lie on your back and lift your legs in a flutter motion. Lift at the desired height in order to keep your lower back pressed to the floor. *Level 3:* Lift your upper body and tuck your chin. Breathe constantly.

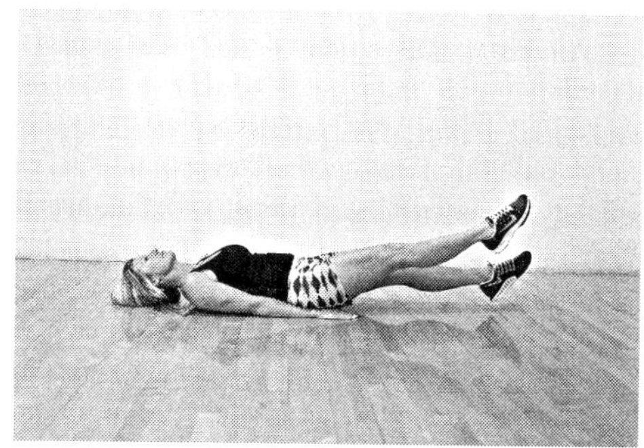

23. *Flutter Taps/Squats:* Stand upright, hop with your feet and land with your right foot in front of the other. Immediately repeat so the left leg leads. While the left leg is ready to switch again, jump right back out and perform a squat. Repeat and lead with the left leg. Keep legs somewhat straight in the air during your flutter. The move should be close to the ground with a small little flutter jump. *Level 1 (Taps):* Take out the jump and tap with your right leg in the front and then the left, then step out to a squat.

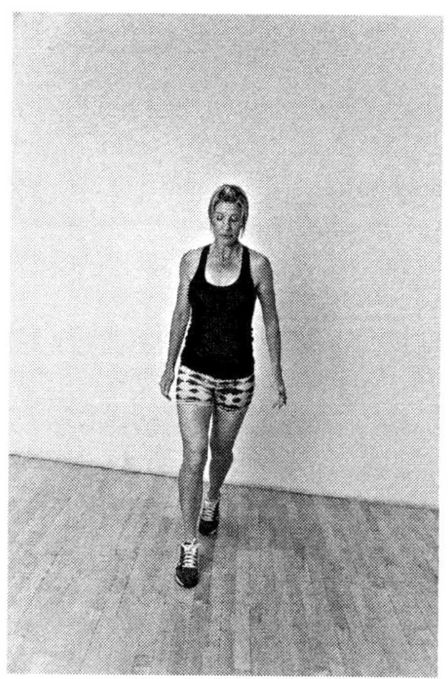
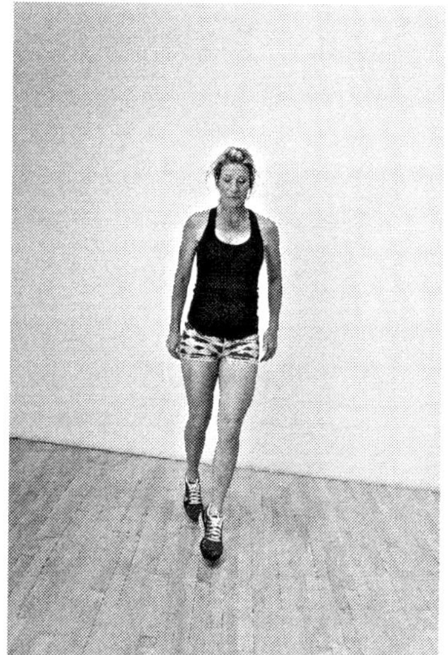
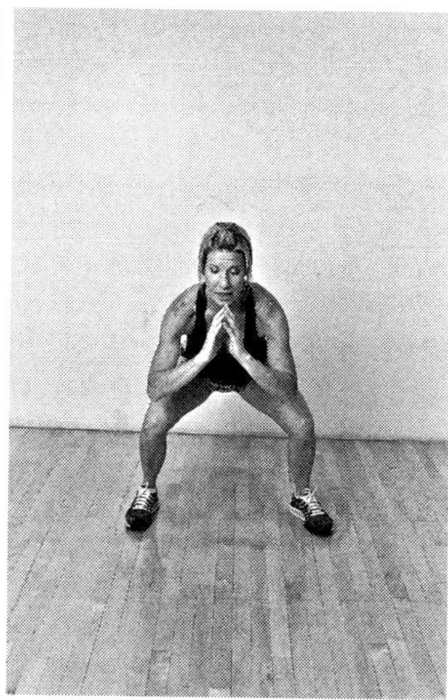

24. *Flye Crunches:* This exercise is two in one. Follow the same directions in Flyes, but keep your core engaged and add a crunch while bringing your arms together. You can either keep your legs straight or bent as needed. Pay attention to your lower back and keep it flat on the floor.

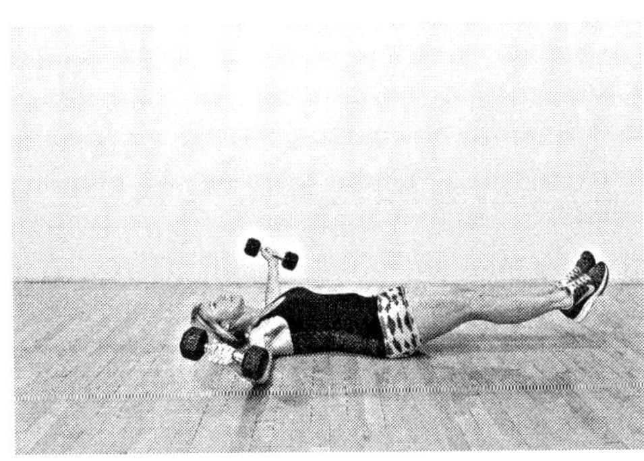

25. *Flyes:* Lie on your back, knees bent, push your lower back into the floor. Take light to medium hand weights straight up and over the center of your chest, not over your chin. Keep a slight bend in your elbows and inhale as you lower them slowly out to the side in a 'T' position. Bracing your core, squeeze your armpits together and exhale as you bring your arms back to the starting position. Squeeze your elbows together as you lift for added intensity **Sometimes you will feel this exercise the day after and not so much while performing it. For this reason, start off with a smaller weight than you would think. It is very important never to straighten your elbows.*

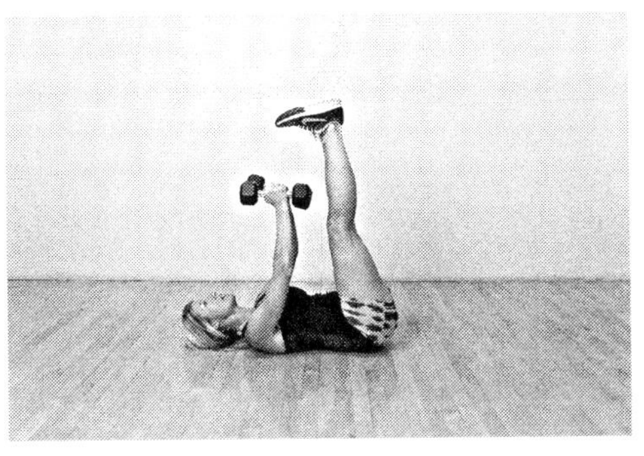

26. *Goblet Squat:* Similar to Plie Squat except take a heavier weight and do not lift your heels off the ground.

27. *Gorilla Jumps:* Jump with your arms over your head and immediately squat and touch the ground. Keep your chest high without dropping it below your hips. Keep your knees behind your toes. Immediately repeat this exercise.

28. *Hammer Curl:* Similar to bicep curl, but turn your hands so your fingers face each other. Slowly curl alternating arms all the way up close to the shoulder and all the way back down close to the thighs. Keep elbows locked by your sides, only bending them, but not moving them.

29. *Hamstring Bridge on Stability Ball:* Lie on the floor on your back. Using a stability ball, place heels near the center of the ball and rest your calves on the ball as well. The ball should be touching your rear end. Slowly lift your hips off the ground while keeping your legs on the ball. Slowly bring them down. Repeat this motion. Brace your core. If you feel too much pressure in the back of your knees, bring the ball closer to your rear and do not lift as high.

30. *Handstand Kick Up/Push Ups:* Start in a plank position, kick your legs up to a handstand and then immediately come back down to a plank position. While in the plank, perform a push up. Switch legs and kick up again to repeat the exercise. *Level 1:* Kick up one leg at a time to become used to inverting your body. This is a huge cardio output exercise, especially when performed quickly. Come up slowly when finished with the exercise, as you can easily become light-headed. *Level 3:* Push up in the handstand is optional.

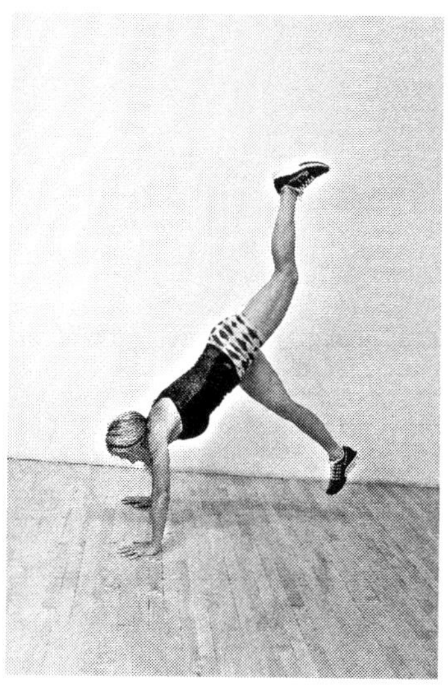

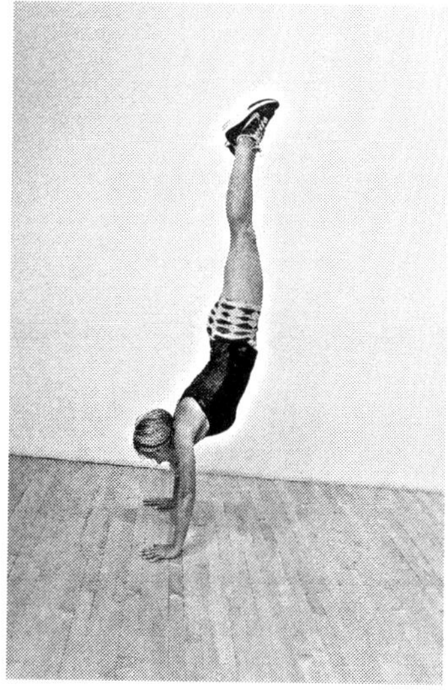

31. *High Knees:* Jog in place while getting your knees up as high and as you can. Keep your core braced and land lightly on the balls of your feet.

32. *Hot Potato:* Lie on your left side, take your right leg and tap it out in front of you on the floor two times, and then behind you on the floor two times. Repeat on other side.

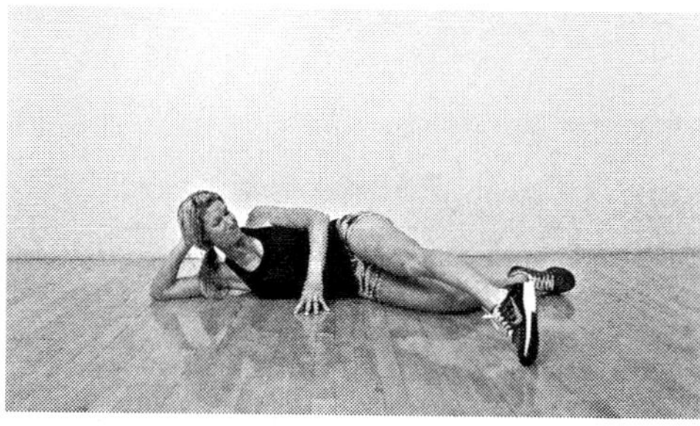

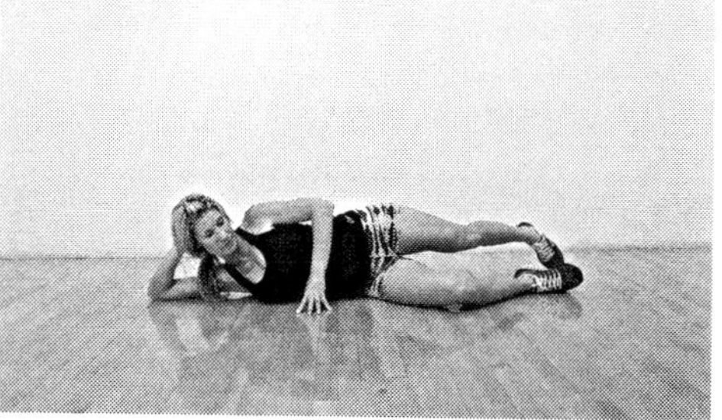

33. *Inner Thighs:* Lie on your left side, bend your right leg and place your right foot close on the floor behind you. Take your left leg and flex your foot while you lift it up and down. Only lift as high as it feels comfortable. If you point and flex your foot, it will add intensity. Keep your neck relaxed and your core braced.

34. *Jogging Rear Kickers:* Jog in place while kicking your heels to your rear.

35. *L-Crunch:* In a crunch position on your back, cross your right ankle over the left knee. Raise your slightly bent left leg up and down (right leg is along for the ride). Breathe in as you lift and out as you let your leg down without touching the ground. Switch legs after designated reps. *Level 1:* Slightly bend left leg to keep your lower back on the ground. *Level 3:* Try to keep leg somewhat straight for added difficulty.

36. *Lat Pull-Downs:* Perform this exercise using an exercise machine.

37. *Lateral Shoulder Raise:* Stand tall with core engaged and slowly raise slightly bent arms out to the side in a 'T' motion. Never lift arms above shoulder height. Slowly release with the same speed back to the beginning position. Repeat.

38. *Lateral Shuffle Hop:* Take two shuffle steps sideways and then add a hop with your arms reaching overhead as high as you can. Then, touch the ground with your hands while in a low squat with your chest lifted high. Then immediately shuffle back the other way. Repeat as quickly as possible back and forth.

39. *Lateral Walking Squats With Bands:* Secure a circle band around your calves or ankles and walk sideways in a deep squat. Keep your knees behind your toes and chest lifted. Keep your hips back and down. If you feel it more in your hips, the band is either too strong or you need to squat deeper. This should target your muscles in your inner and outer thighs, your glutes, and your quads.

40. *Leg Raises:* On your back, in crunch position with knees bent and back pressed to the ground, slowly drop one leg down towards the ground while keeping the other bent over your hip. Slowly switch legs continuously.

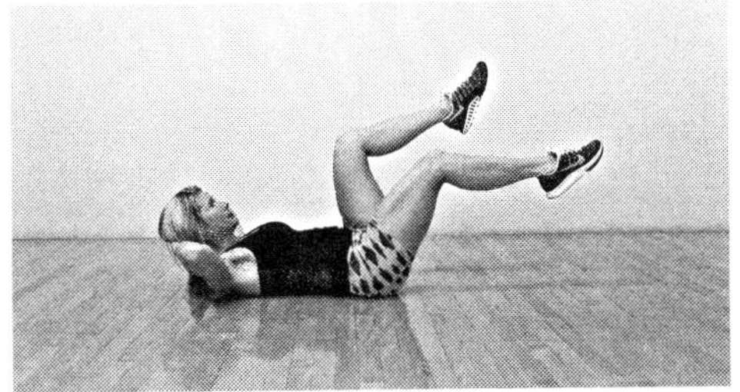

41. *Lunge/Pulses:* In a lunge position, one leg forward and one leg back, both bending, keep front knee behind your front toes. Put pressure in your front heel and not your toes. Do not let your back knee touch the floor. Only go as low as your flexibility allows. *Pulses:* In a lunge position, slightly pulse up and down—only a few inches each way.

42. *Lying Leg Lifts:* Lie on your right side in a slight half-moon position. Take your left leg and lift it as high as feels comfortable. You can take your knee and face the ceiling or face it forward. Lower with the same speed you lifted. Keep your core braced and your neck relaxed. Repeat on the other side.

43. *Mountain Climbers:* In a plank position and arms straight, bend one knee and take it to your chest, while keeping your hips low and bracing your core. Then, switch to the other leg. You can hop with this motion quickly, or tap one foot at a time.

44. *Oblique Lifts:* Lie on your right side, in a slight half-moon position, lift both your legs together and brace yourself with your left hand if needed on the ground in front of you. Engaging your obliques and inner and outer thighs, either pulse or lift your legs up and down. Try to lift your legs higher than your hips. Breathe constantly while you perform this exercise.

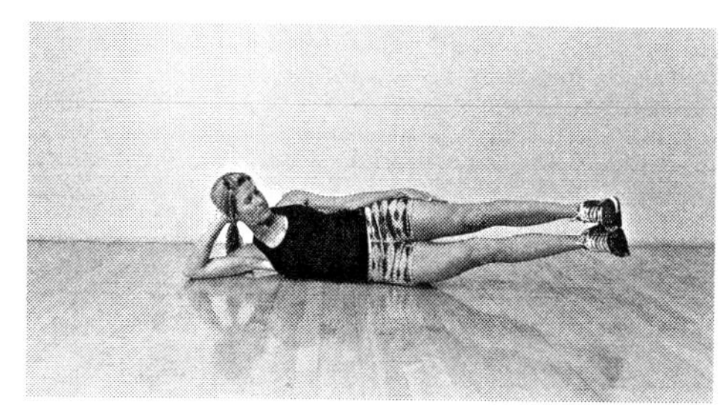

45. *Plank:* In a plank position, either using extended arms or resting on your elbows, position your body like a straight board—a plank. Most execute this incorrectly because their rear end is too high or too low. It should look like one straight line from your head to your toes. You can modify and drop to your knees at any time. Make sure your shoulders are right over your elbows. Breathe in and out slowly as you contract your bottom and legs and hold the exercise. **Level 3:** To make this more difficult, pull or draw your hips towards your shoulder and squeeze with a slight rotation in your hips towards your elbows. Brace your core and draw in your navel.

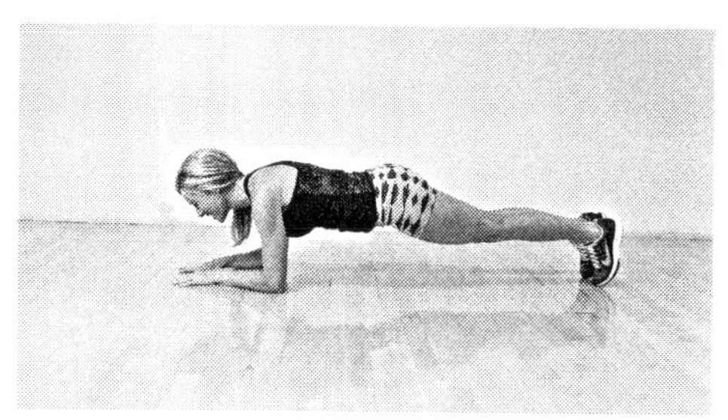

46. *Plank High Fives:* With a partner if possible (or use the air), start in a plank position with arms extended off your elbows. Face your partner and place yourself about an arms distance away. Give each other a high five using your opposite hands back and forth. Try to clap about shoulder height for intensity. Maintain a plank position throughout the exercise. *Level 1:* Instead of a full plank, go to your knees.

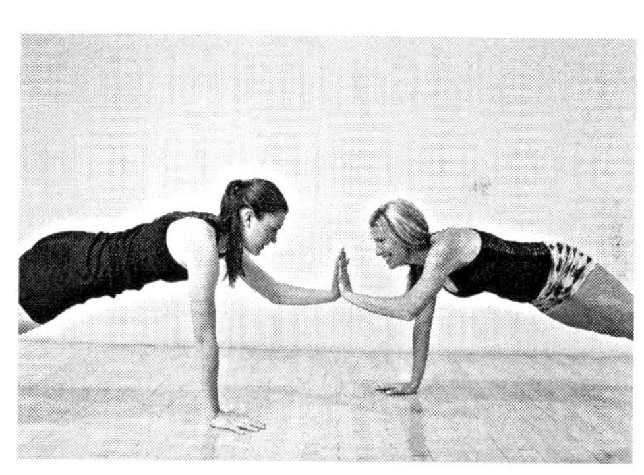

47. *Plank Knees to Elbow:* In a plank position, arms extended, bring in one knee towards your opposite elbow and then return back to starting position. Repeat on other leg. Keep hips low in a plank position throughout the exercise.

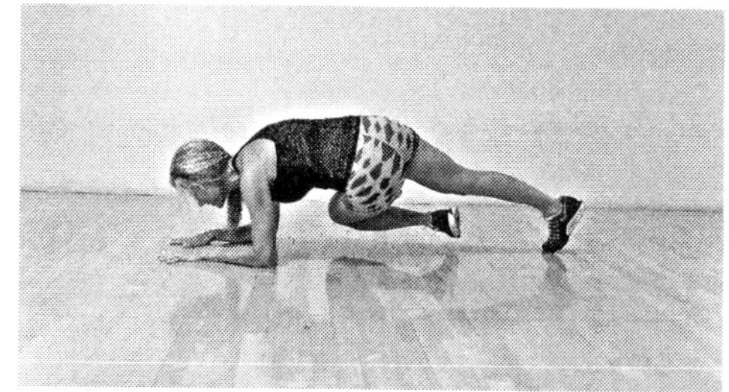

48. *Plank Middle Hip Dips:* In a plank position on your elbows, slowly twist your hips side to side. Do not feel like you have to touch the floor with your hips. Rather, think about the muscles being used. Breathe constantly in and out. If this exercise irritates your back, perform a plank instead.

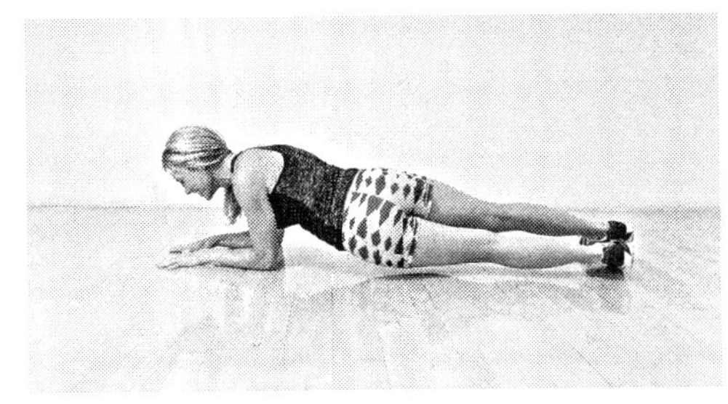

49. *Plank Tappers/Hoppers:* In a plank position, preferably with extended arms, take one leg slightly out and tap it to the ground lightly. Then return it to the beginning position. Repeat with the other leg to its own side. Repeat. *Level 3:* Hop both feet out at the same time and then back again while remaining in a plank. You can extend arms or perform on your elbows. This exercise can strain the back easily if not performing it with light hops. Please only hop if you have a strong back. If you have lower back issues, please try a basic plank or a crunch instead.

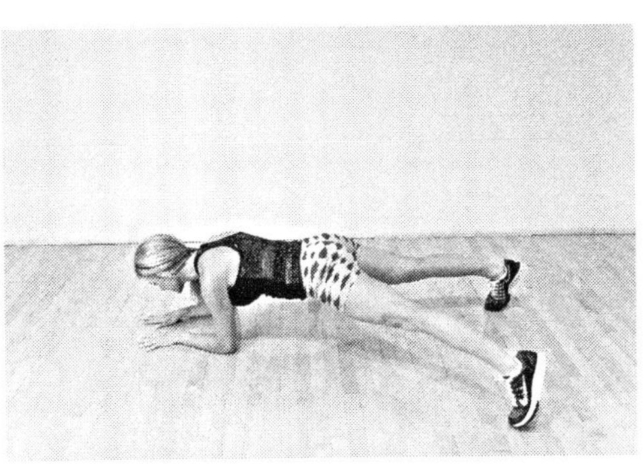

50. *Plate Sliders:* Stand in a lunge with your left leg in the back. Use a hardy paper plate or furniture slider on carpet, or nylon socks on hardwood floor under your back left foot. Slowly slide the leg to a full standing position and then slide the plate back to the lunge. *Level 1:* Hold on to a handrail or furniture to make sure you don't overextend.

51. *Plie Squats:* Position yourself so you are in a very wide squat with toes facing out slightly. Your knees should track with your toes and it should feel natural with no pain in your knees. Keep your chest tall and squat, then come back up. *Levels 2 & 3:* Lift one or both heels in the air for added intensity.

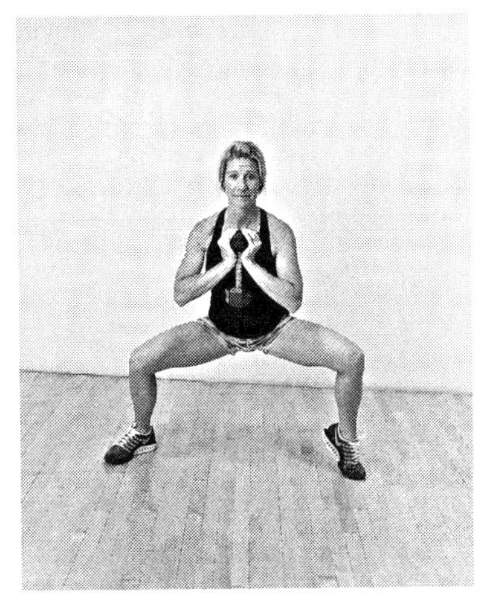

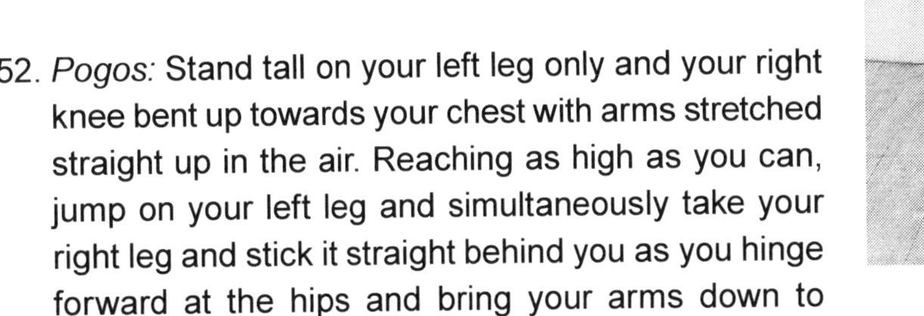

52. *Pogos:* Stand tall on your left leg only and your right knee bent up towards your chest with arms stretched straight up in the air. Reaching as high as you can, jump on your left leg and simultaneously take your right leg and stick it straight behind you as you hinge forward at the hips and bring your arms down to touch the floor. Repeat with the same leg and sequence for designated reps. *Level 1:* Take out the hop and do not worry about trying to touch the floor, just reach as

far as you can. If you become dizzy, do not go as fast or down as low. You do not have to touch the floor.

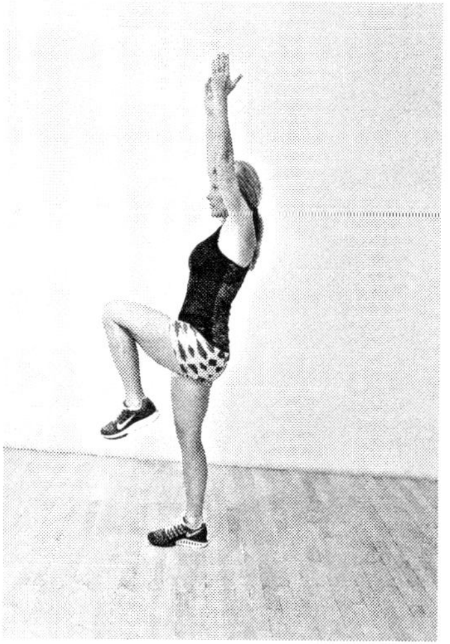

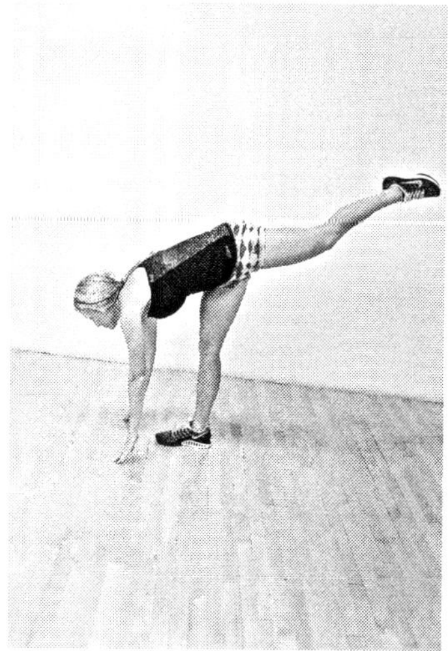

53. *Potatoes*: Lie on the floor on one side, head comfortably laying on your arm or hand with elbow bent, raise your top leg while keeping your knee facing forward, and tap it two times in the front—keeping it straight—and then tap it two times in the back. Keep your hips stacked during this exercise. Try not to lean forward when tapping the front. Repeat.

54. *Prisoner Squats/Kicks/Hops: Squats:* Take your hands and place them behind your head, like a surrender position. Squat with knees behind the toes with weight in the heels. Stand straight up and push through the heels. Keep hands behind head to increase heart rate. You can drop your hands if it is too difficult. *Kicks:* As you squat and come back up, kick one leg forward then go back to a squat. Repeat on the other leg. *Hops:* Add a hop at the bottom of the squat. Keep knees soft and your hands tucked behind your head in a prisoner position.

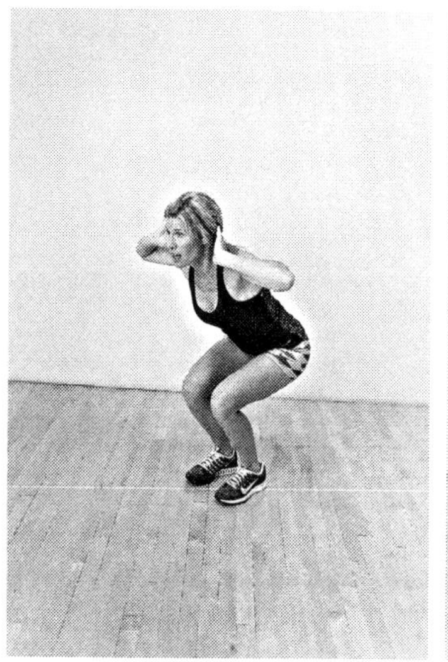

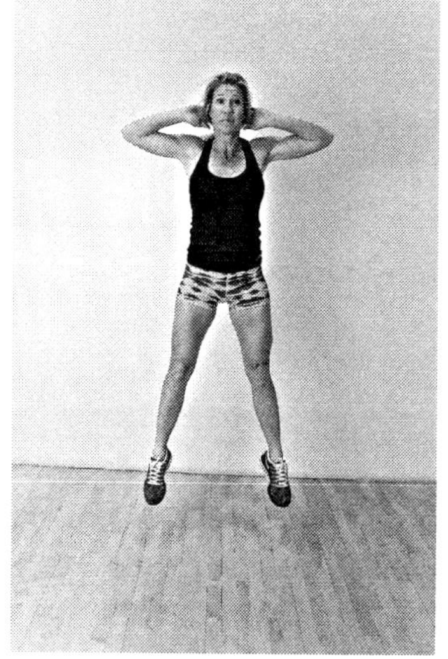

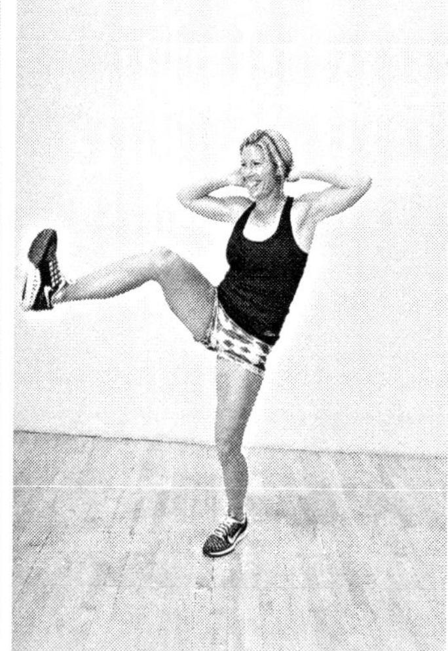

55. *Rainbows:* Lie on your left side and take your right leg and bend it. Swing it out in front of you with a large arch motion—like a rainbow. Tap the floor with your knee and then reverse your leg and touch the floor with your foot (not your knee) behind you. Keep your neck neutral and core engaged.

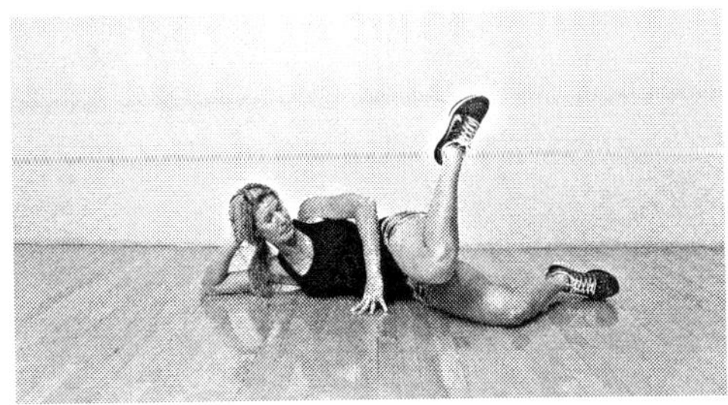

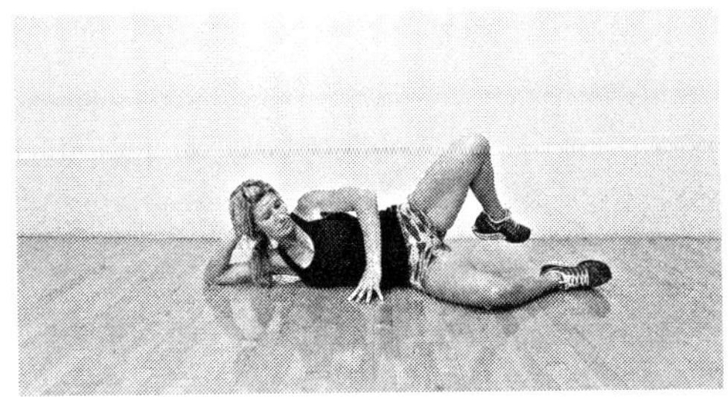

56. *Reverse Crunch:* Lie on your back, press it to the ground, and bring your legs straight up over your hips. Slightly lift your bottom off the ground and then back again. Try to go as high as you can with your legs as you lift with force and back down quickly. Think about holding a bag of flour on your flexed feet. Try not to drop the bag of flour. Control the motion. *Level 1:* Lift slowly and controlled using the same speed going up and down.

57. *Reverse Flyes:* Lean over in a lunge, hinging at the hips. Keep knees behind the front toes. Draw in your abs and keep knees soft and bent. Slightly bend elbows and blow air out as you extend your arms out to the sides in a 'T' motion. Never raise higher than your shoulders. You should focus on being able to see your arms at all times. Squeeze your lower shoulder blades together as you lift. **If you have back issues, do not attempt this exercise.*

58. *Reverse Lunges:* In a lunge position, prop your back leg up on a small stool or step. Perform a lunge by bending your front straight leg. Your back leg will naturally bend slightly. You will feel this in many areas of your lower body. Keep your chest tall and your core braced. This will challenge your balance if you do not hold on to anything.

59. *Roman Walks:* Reach out with your right arm and kick up your left leg as straight as possible and try to reach for your toes. Then bring your arm and foot back to the beginning position. Repeat with the other arm and leg. Keep this sequence going as you slightly move forward with each step.

60. *Scorpions: Level 3:* An advanced exercise or for those with a stronger back. In a plank position, on your elbows, bend left knee and reach your left leg over the right hip and tap the floor. Maintain plank position and keep elbows connected with the floor at all times. Repeat on the other side. If you cannot touch the floor at the beginning, keep working at it.

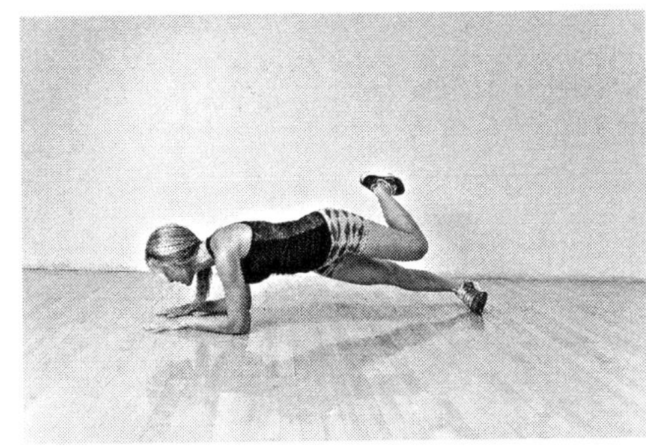

61. *Seal Crunches:* Starting on your back or with shoulder blades slightly lifted, pull yourself up to a crunch position while taking your hands towards your toes. Keep chin tucked and end on your bottom only. Reverse this position and immediately perform again.

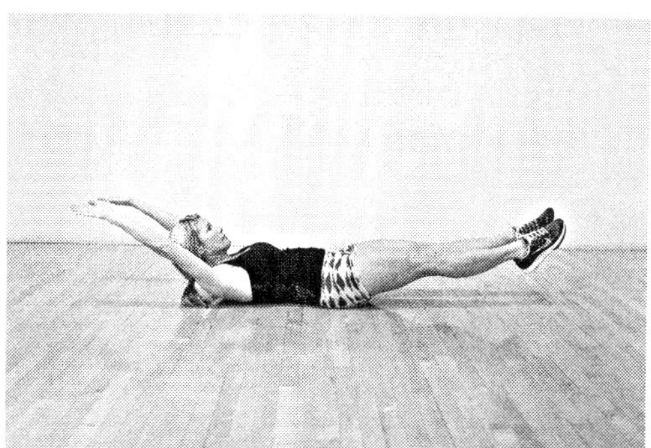

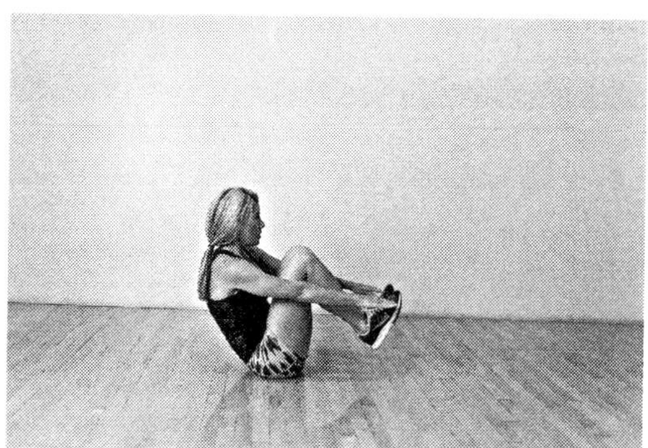

62. *Seated Rows:* This is a rowing exercise to be performed sitting at an exercise machine.

63. *Side Lunges:* Once you have mastered the regular lunge, you can take it up a notch. Start by standing in a wide stance, legs straight and much wider than your hips. Squat with only one leg and keep the other straight with weight in your squatted leg. Push through your heel as you stand up with straight wide legs. Keep chest lifted and core braced. Repeat.

64. *Side Plank Dips:* In a side elbow plank, with feet in scissors or knees together, lift your hips and push them slightly forward so your body looks like one straight line (including your neck and head). Once in a good starting plank position, dip your hips towards the ground and then up to towards the ceiling. **If this irritates your back or shoulder, or is too hard on your sides (obliques), take it down to a knee, dip slightly, or hold it in a side plank. Slowly build up to a more advanced move, or just skip this exercise.*

65. *Side Plank Thread the Needle:* In a left side plank position, on your elbow, turn your shoulders and hips towards the ground and thread your right arm under your chest. Touch the floor behind you if you can. Then go back to the starting side position. Repeat.

66. *Single Leg Reverse Lunge:* This exercise begins in a lunge, except you take your back leg and prop it up on your toes, a stool, a bench, or a step. You choose the height of your apparatus. Lunge as normal with the pressure in your front heel. Keep your front knee behind your toes. You do not want to feel this primarily in your hip flexor; rather you want to feel it in your legs. Think of your back leg as the primary focus. Your front leg is along for the ride by only bending it, not moving it forward or back. *Level 1:* Begin with a regular lunge before taking it to a raised level behind you.

67. *Skaters:* Begin with a jump, landing with back leg in a curtsey position while swinging one arm in the air and the other towards the floor (see photo). Immediately hop to the other side. Keep head looking in the same direction of the bottom arm. *Level 1:* Take out the hop and just tap curtsey lunges with arm swings side to side.

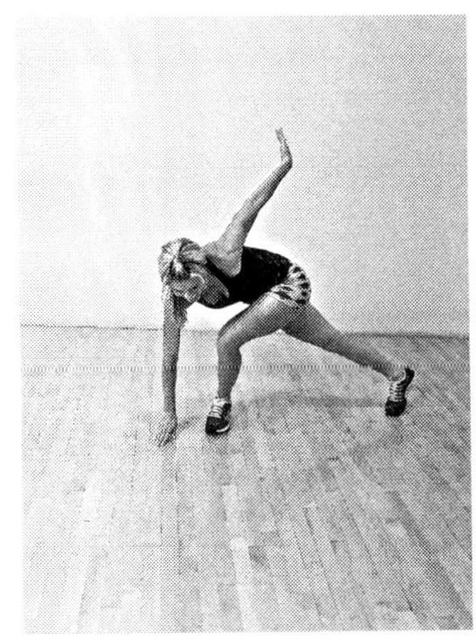

68. *Squat Thrusts:* This is the same exercise as the Burpee, except you do not jump with your hands overhead at the top. Perform a squat and then head to the ground and thrust your body into a plank position. As soon as you hit the plank, immediately come back up and then back into a squat. Repeat.

69. *Standing Band Leg Raises:* In a semi-squatted position, with a band around your calves, pulse or lift one leg off to the side and then back. You can do this without a band for lesser intensity. Go slowly and brace your core. Keep your chest lifted high.

70. *Star Crunches: Level 2-3:* Lie on your back, extend your arms and legs out in an 'X' position. Slowly bring up your legs and shoot your arms through your legs while crunching up with your chest. You can come as high as you'd like—moving while keeping your back on the ground or lift your back off the floor and all the way up in a sit up position.

71. *Star Jumps:* Start in a squat position, propel your body forward and swing your arms in the air at the same time into an 'X' overhead, then back to a squatting position, landing with soft knees. Repeat as fast as you can. *Level 1 (Leg Lifts):* If you cannot jump, take one leg and same arm out to the side (side leg lift), and then squat back down to this starting position before doing the same thing on the other side.

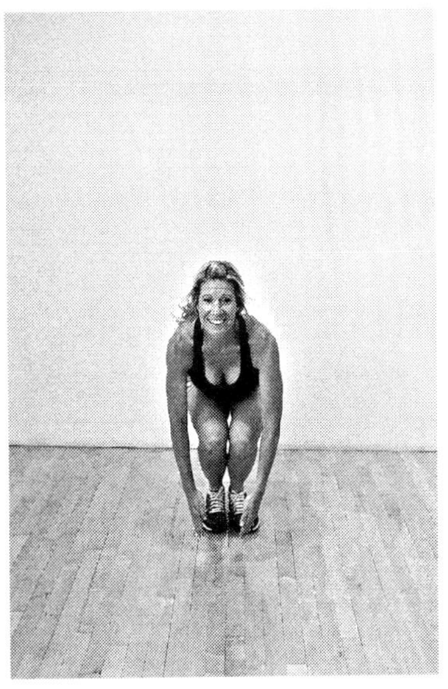

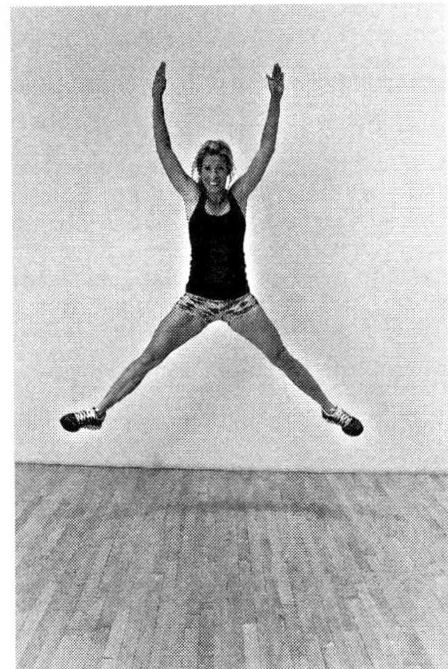

72. *Stationary Backward Lunges:* Stand with feet close together, step back into a lunge. Keep the front knee behind the front toes. Dip your back knee close to the floor and then come back to a standing position with legs close together. Switch legs and repeat. Go slowly and brace your core. Keep your chest lifted high.

73. *Stationary Football Run:* Jog in place as fast as you can and keep your feet super low to the ground, like a light stomping motion but on the balls of your feet only. The higher your knees come toward your chest, the more you engage your core. Use your arms to increase your speed and increase your cardio output.

74. *Sumo Side Kicks:* Stand in a squatted sumo position (legs wide, toes slightly turned out, hips back, knees behind your toes with your chest lifted) and kick one leg to the side without extending it fully. Remain in a squatted lower position while kicking and then go back to the sumo squat. Repeat on the other side.

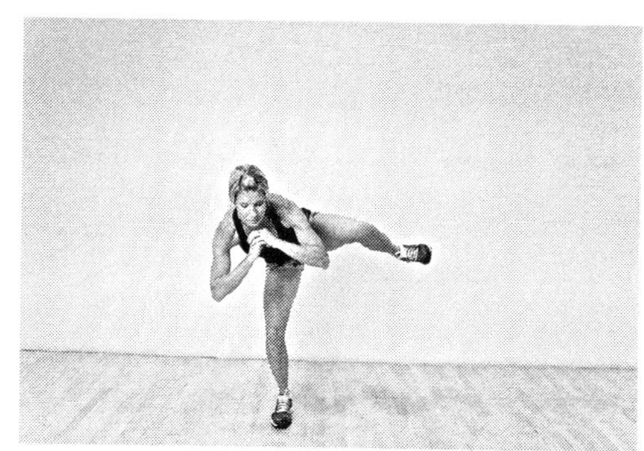

75. *Surfers:* Lie flat on your stomach in a "Swimmer" position (arms and legs off the ground). Lift your legs and arms in a swimming motion up and down for 2-5 seconds before quickly getting up and jumping into a low squat. Quickly reverse by getting back down to the starting position. **Option to just perform swimmer, first photo, without getting up.*

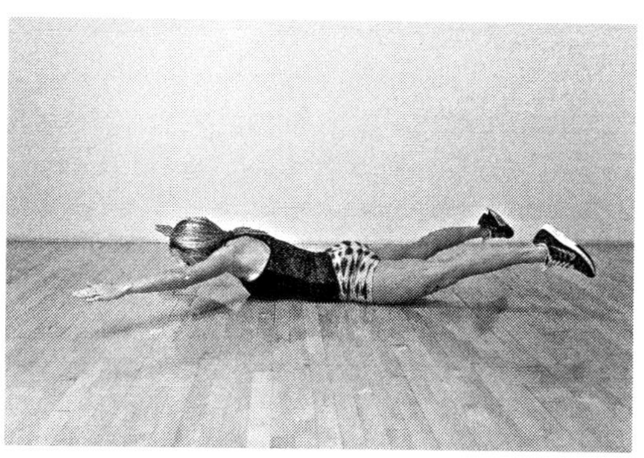

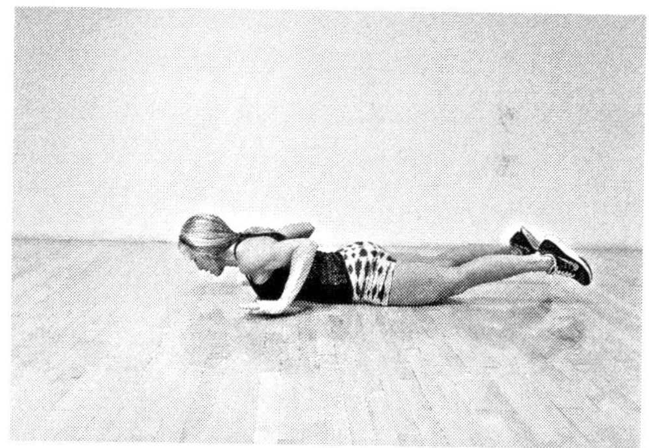

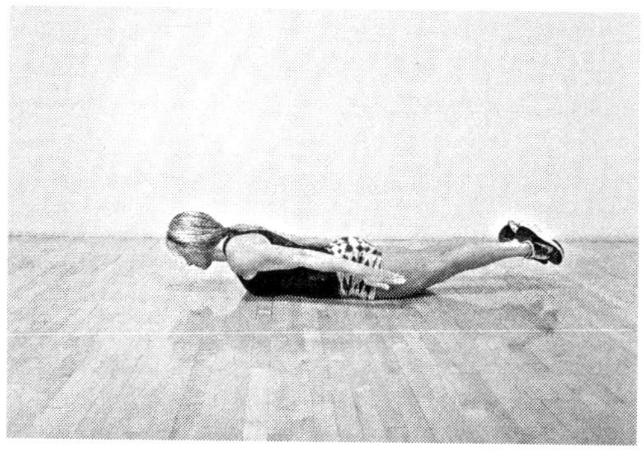

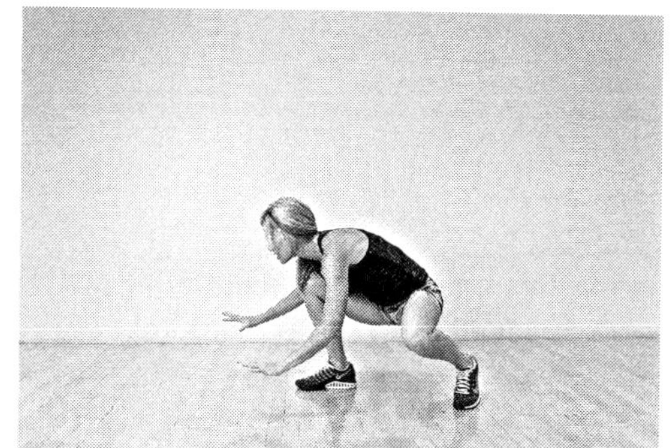

76. *Swimmers:* Lie flat on your stomach in a full-body stretch with palms down touching the ground. Slowly raise your arms and legs a few inches off the ground. Keep eyes focused on the ground with your neck neutral. Move your arms and legs as if you were swimming—in a flutter motion. *Level 1:* Keep legs or arms down to make it easier.

77. *Switch Taps/Squats:* Similar to the Flutter Squats but instead of tapping or hopping to the front, tap or cross your legs across your body in the front with one or both legs at a time.

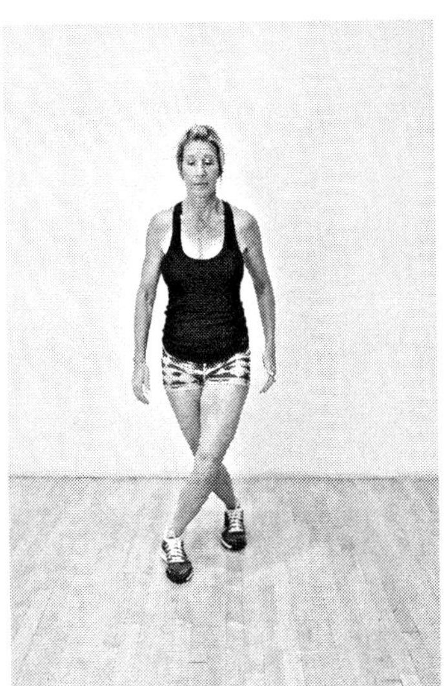

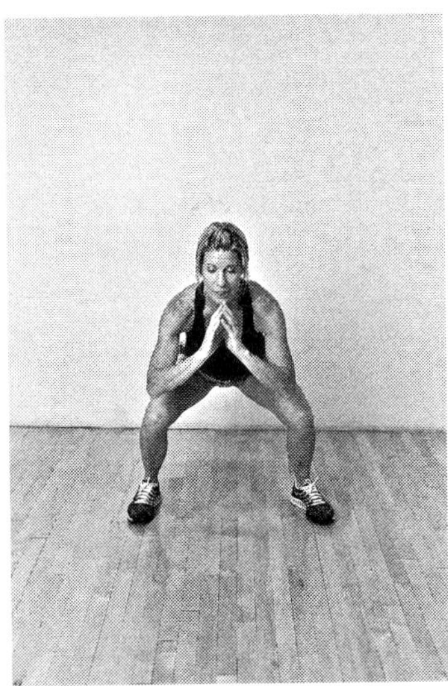

78. *Triceps Dips:* Use the floor or any type of support (chair, table, counter, stool), place hands on the edge, fingertips facing your bottom. Keep your bottom as close as you can to the support. Slowly lower yourself down a few inches. Keep elbows facing behind you as you squeeze them together. Make your body weight evenly distributed while keeping your chest high. Try not to dip lower than 90 degrees with your elbows. **If you have bad shoulders or elbows, do not attempt this exercise. Try Triceps Extension or Triceps Kickback instead.*

79. *Triceps Extension:* Raise a light/moderate weight overhead with hands clasped together and squeeze. Draw in your abs for support. Bending your elbows, slowly lower the weight down as close to the nape of your neck as you can while squeezing elbows in. Then raise it to the starting position. **If you do not feel it in your triceps by rep 8, squeeze elbows together more at the top and bottom of the exercise, or choose a heavier weight.*

80. *Triceps Kickback:* Bend over at the hips, knees slightly bent. Pull in abs and squeeze elbows to your sides with bent arms (weights by chest), fingers facing in. Lock your elbows to your sides and do not move them, except bending only. Kick back to almost straight arms (keep a slight bend). Then return to starting position. **If you do not feel this in your triceps by rep 8, then lean forward more, make sure elbows are not moving, or use a heavier weight.*

81. *Tuck Jumps: Level 3:* Stand upright and jump high with your knees as close to your hips and stomach as possible. Land softly on the balls of your feet and repeat as fast as possible. Keep chest high and core braced.

82. *Twisters:* Lie on your back in crunch position. Lift your lower body off the ground like the Reverse Crunch, but slightly bend your knees and bring them somewhat close to your chest. Swing your knees side to side in a twisting motion. Focus on your obliques. *Level 1:* Keep your head and shoulders on the ground.

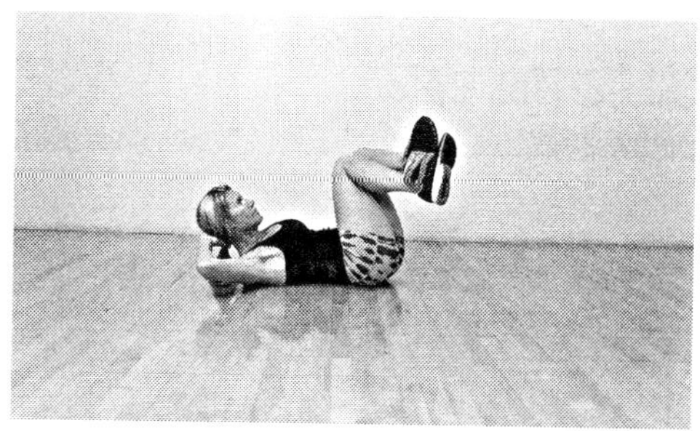

83. *YTWL:* Lie on your stomach and slightly raise your head, neck, and shoulders. Keep palms facing down for the entire exercise. Hold arms in a 'Y', then to a 'T', then to a 'W', and then to an 'L' and repeat. Keep eyes down and neck neutral and look at the mat the entire time.

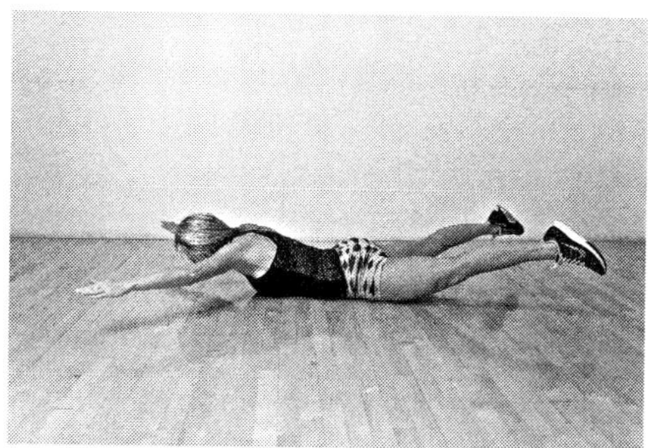

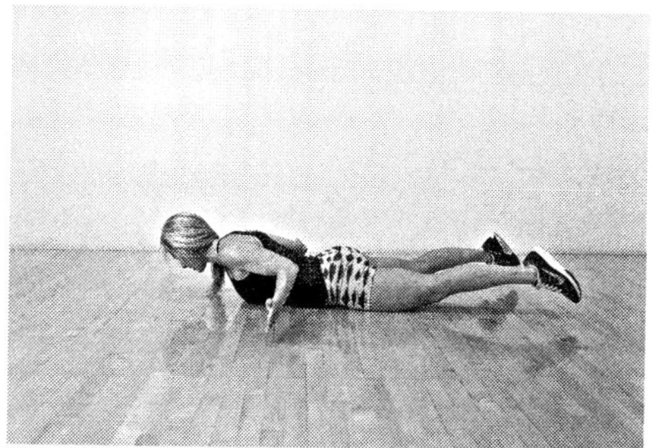

MEAL PLANNING

MEAL PLANNING STEP 1: IDENTIFY YOUR REAL CONSUMPTION

Meal Plan Levels

Just as we have different levels of exercise, we have various levels of nutrition. Decide which level you are right now. Aim to progress in nutrition as you continue with your goals.

Level 1	Level 2	Level 3
Beginner	**Intermediate**	**Advanced**
—New to meal planning	—Familiar with meal planning	—Strict meal planning
—Crave foods all the time	—Little knowledge about personal eating	—Understands/eats organics regularly
—Possible eating disorder	—Attempts diet plans	—Solid nutrition, a way of life
—Can't control eating	—Yo-yo eating patterns	—Can control cravings
—Needing to clean up eating now	Weight to lose	No weight to lose

We all choose about 20-30 foods and rotate through them on a regular basis. When we go to the store, we tend to stick to the same brands as well. Much like when we go out to eat, we settle for one of the top five favorites. We are creatures of habit! Not a bad thing, but it could be if the habits are not that healthy.

1. **Be honest and record 20-30 breakfast, snack, lunch, and dinner foods that you eat on a regular basis (record brand names if possible).** See Sarah's list on the next page for examples.

2. **Circle all the packaged food items: yogurt, protein bars and powders, crackers, chips, string cheese, lunchmeat, TV dinners, etc.**

Cheat Sheet – Sarah's Basic Foods

These are foods I eat most often for breakfast, snack, lunch, and dinner, and the brand names and where I purchase them. Some brands or options can come and go. The point is to know where your food comes from and what is in it.

1. Organic vegetables—sweet potatoes, broccoli, carrots, celery, spinach, kale, onions, peppers, mushrooms
2. Free range eggs—local Engelbrecht Farmers
3. Old fashioned oatmeal—Quaker
4. Organic green tea and coffee—Bromley, or other
5. Organic half & half—Organic Valley
6. Organic fruits—apples, bananas, peaches, pears, berries, oranges, grapefruits, melons, pineapple *(I can't always find or purchase organic)*
7. Skim cottage cheese—Organic Valley
8. Plain Greek yogurt—Stoneybrook and Organic Valley
9. Popcorn—air popped
10. Local raw honey—local farmer or local grocery store
11. Nuts—almonds & walnuts, plain and unsalted
12. Quinoa—Ancient Harvest
13. Rice—brown, long grain, jasmine
14. Beef—local VonMuenster Farm
15. Tuna—packed in water
16. Organic or grass-fed butter—Organic Valley, or local
17. Milled Flax—Hodgson Mill or organic in bulk
18. Unsweetened vanilla almond milk (plus protein)—So Delicious or Silk
19. Rice cakes—Quaker, plain or apple cinnamon
20. Corn tortilla chips—On the Border and various options
21. Salsa—homemade or various brands
22. Protein bars—Premier Protein, Nature Valley Peanut, with many various options
23. Spices—cinnamon, nutmeg, basil, oregano, turmeric, salt, pepper, rosemary, cumin, dill; from my garden or health food store options

MEAL PLANNING STEP 2: GET A GRIP ON THE FOOD LABEL

Since I do not exactly know what brands of foods you enjoy most, here are the *general guidelines* to see if at least 75% of your 20-30 basic foods are healthy. Use the footnote at the bottom of the label to reference your daily intake requirements of your 20-30 basic foods choices.

1. **Food Selection:** Take a packaged food that you eat most often (something in a bag or container) and identify the following:
    a. How many calories are in this food choice per serving?
    b. Do you typically only eat one serving size? (If not, add your intake accordingly.)
2. **Limit:** Saturated fats should be under 20 grams total for the day, if you consume 2000 calories. Never consume trans fats.
3. **Consume Enough:** When we eat on the run we tend to not consume enough vital nutrients. This is when it is a good idea to take a multivitamin (from a reputable source).
4. **Use the footnote:** Compare your overall daily totals to the total on the packaged food, then aim to make yours close to the footnote.
5. **General Rule:** If your food label reads under 5% in the far right column, it is generally too low. If it reads 20% or more, it is too high. (*It takes us back to Goldilocks—balance it out, so it is just right.)*

Nutrition Facts

2 servings per container
Serving Size 1 cup (228g)

Amount per serving	
Calories	**250**
	% Daily Value*
Total Fat 12g	
Saturated Fat 3g	15%
Trans Fat 3g	
Cholesterol 30mg	10%
Sodium 470mg	20%
Total Carbohydrates 31g	10%
Dietary Fiber 0g	0%
Total Sugars 5g	
Includes 0g Added Sugars	20%
Protein 5g	
Vitamin D 2mcg	10%
Calcium 260mg	20%
Iron 8mg	45%
Potassium 235mg	6%

* The % Daily Value (DV) tells you how much a nutrient in a serving of food contributes to a daily diet. 2,000 calories a day is used for general nutrition advice.

6. **Added Sugar:** How much added sugar is in your food?
7. **Remember:** The average woman should not consume more than 20 grams of added sugar per day. Added Sugars: sugars naturally not found in foods (fruit does not have added sugar—it is natural). Look at the ingredients list—it will tell you.
8. **Don't Buy:** Try not to purchase foods that contain these ingredients listed first in the food label—bleached flour, sugar, or yeast.
9. **Does Your Food Make The Cut?** Instead of cutting out your type of food, try finding a healthier alternative.

MEAL PLANNING STEP 3: IDENTIFY YOUR CALORIC GOALS

The next 15 minutes could help you find the key to the difference between gaining weight or losing it.

1. Choose a free online calorie counter (myfitnesspal, choosemyplate, loseit), register, and plug in every single thing you consumed (food and drinks) in the past three to four days.
2. Take the average daily calories consumed of those three to four days. My average current daily caloric intake is ________________.
3. Multiply this daily number by seven to obtain your *current* weekly calories. My weekly caloric intake is ________________.
4. To lose one pound per week, you have three options:
    a. Consume 3,500 calories less than your current caloric intake each week.
    b. Burn 3,500 calories with exercise each week.
    c. Consume 1,750 fewer calories and burn 1,750 calories with exercise per week.
    Note: A weight loss of two pounds per week needs 7,000 less calories.

5. The best way to figure how many calories you burn during exercise is to wear a heart rate monitor. It must be set up with your age, weight, height, and resting heart rate to obtain a good reading. *Some HRM's do not give a number of calories burned with exercise, so please check before purchasing. An average one-hour fitness class can burn about 500 calories.
6. Fill in: I want to lose ________________ pounds. It will take me ________________ weeks.
7. My new weekly caloric intake will be ________________ (with reduced food and exercise).
8. Divide your new weekly caloric intake by seven, and you will have your new daily intake: ________________.

Please follow the important safety guidelines for losing weight. Do not consume under 1200 calories per day or aim to lose more than 2 pounds per week unless under the care and advisement of your physician. If you are uncertain of your caloric needs, please see a local professional for help.

Breaking Down Your Calories

This section is about getting accurate with macronutrients (carbohydrates, proteins, and fats). *Please note, these are general guidelines, and your suggested intakes could be different. If you are unsure of your personal macronutrients needs and breakdowns, please see a local professional.*

Macros and Their Calorie Counterparts	Carbohydrates	Protein	Fats
	4 cal/gram	4 cal/gram	9 cal/gram
Recommended Macro-nutrient by Age			
Young children (1-3 yrs)	45-65%	5-20%	30-40%
Older children and adolescents (4-18 yrs)	45-65%	10-30%	25-35%
Adults (19 yrs +)	45-65%	10-35%	20-35%

Table information provided the FDA.

For easy math, we will use a daily 2,000 caloric intake for our sample.

1. Carbohydrates should constitute 45%-65% of our total consumption. If you want to lose weight aggressively, you could strive for 45% carbs; if you are not trying to lose weight, you could strive up to 65% carbs.

2. Protein should constitute 10%-35% of your total intake. If you engage in intense sports or performance/weight lifting programs, your protein intake could increase. Protein intake is calculated on body weight (generally .4 x lb or 1 x lb—many differing suggestions).

3. Fats should constitute 25-30% of total intake. Remember, we are supposed to consume *healthy* fats.

MEAL PLANNING STEP 4: CHOOSING WISELY

Vegetables & Fruit

Circle all the vegetables and fruits you will eat. There are over 200 different varieties of fruits and vegetables with all the different color choices.

Vegetables

Red	beets, red bell pepper, radish, tomato, red onion, rhubarb
Orange/Yellow	yellow beet, butternut & yellow & winter squash, carrot, yellow pepper, yellow potato, pumpkin, sweet corn, sweet potato, yellow tomato
Green	artichoke, arugula, asparagus, broccoli, Brussels sprout, Chinese cabbage, green bean, green cabbage, celery, chayote squash, cucumber, endive, edamame, leafy green, leek, lettuce, green onion, okra, pea, green pepper, snow pea, spinach, sugar snap pea, watercress, zucchini
Blue/Violet	black olive, purple asparagus, purple cabbage, purple carrot, egg plant, purple potatoes
White/Brown	cauliflower, garlic, ginger, mushroom, onion, parsnip, white potato, shallots, turnips, white corn, lentil, soybean

Fruits

Red	red apple, blood orange, cherry, cranberry, red grape, pink/red grapefruit, red pear, pomegranate, raspberry, strawberry, watermelon
Orange/Yellow	yellow apple, apricot, cape gooseberry, cantaloupe, yellow fig, grapefruit, golden kiwi, lemon, mango, nectarine, orange, papaya, peach, yellow pear, persimmon, pineapple, tangerine, yellow watermelon
Green	avocado, green apple, honeydew, kiwi, lime
Blue/Violet	blackberry, blueberry, concord grape, dried plum, elderberry, purple fig, purple grape, plum, raisin
White/Brown	banana, date, white nectarine, white peach, brown pear

Proteins & Meats

Below are the most common meat and protein choices. Simply circle the ones you would eat. This is the easiest way to create a healthy meal plan. We do not need too much meat unless we are not getting our protein in other places. It is recommended to consume only about 1.8 ounces of meat per day or 12.6 ounces per week.

Seafood: The FDA recommends eating seafood twice per week for a healthy heart. It is an excellent source of lean protein. Buy local, and it will save you money.

Anchovies	Mackerel	Scallop
Catfish	Mullet	Shrimp
Clam	Oyster	Sole
Crab	Perch	Squid
Crawfish	Pollock	Tilapia
Flounder	Salmon	Trout
Haddock	Sardine	Whitefish
Herring		

Beef: Grass-fed beef is preferred—it is pricey, but worth it for believed healthier components. Depending on your budget, aim for extra lean meat.

Steak Cuts	*Roast Cuts*
Rib-eye	*Chuck Roast*
Fillet	*Rib Roast*
Loin	*Sirloin Roast*
T-Bone	*Round Roast*
Skirt	*Ground Beef*
Flank	*Hamburger*

Prime - fattiest cut
Choice - moderate in fat
Select - leanest grade

Lamb: A staple in Mediterranean diets, lamb is believed to be the world's healthiest meat because of its ability to lower the risk of cardiovascular disease. Lean chops can be as low as 150 calories and 5.6 grams of fat.

 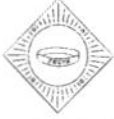

Venison/Deer: Deer contains more moisture and is generally a learner choice than beef or lamb. The taste gets some getting used to, but seasoning helps.

Deli Meat (processed): There are over 200 different types of processed meats. They are cheaper, but higher in fat and sodium. Studies show they may glue meat together with non-meat additives and emulsions including lips, heart, and stomach.

Whole Meat Cuts/Sliced	*Salami*
Low-Sodium Turkey	*Ham*
Chicken Breast	*Bacon*
Lean Roast Beef	*Sausage*
Processed Meats	*Pepperoni*
Bologna	

Poultry: Grilled, roasted, fried, canned, shaved, shredded, baked. Poultry should be skinned to reduce fat.

Turkey	Sausage Links	Thigh
Shaved Turkey	Turkey Bacon — low sodium	Chicken Sausage
Turkey Steak	Chicken	Leg
Ground Turkey	Shaved Chicken	Ground Chicken
Turkey Dogs	Breast	Chicken Brats/Hot Dogs

Dairy: Organic free-range is preferred. *Grass-fed milk has more Vitamin K.

Milk	Greek	Cheese:
Cow's Milk	Low Fat	Cheddar
Goat's Milk	Plain	Mozzarella
Yogurt	Kefir	Swiss
Butter	Goat	Parmesan
Cottage Cheese — low sodium	Whey (Protein Powders)	Blue Cheese
	Eggs	

Beans, Nuts & Peas: These three options are great sources of protein.

Seeds	Nuts	Peas
Adzuki Beans	*Peanut — dry roasted*	Green Peas
Black Beans	*Soy Nuts*	Snow Peas
Soybeans	*Carob Nuts*	Snap Peas
Anasazi Beans	*Almonds*	Split Peas
Flava Beans	*Walnuts*	Black-eyed Peas
Garbanzo Beans (chickpeas)	*Tree Nuts*	Soy/Tofu
Kidney Beans	*Cashews*	
	Pecans	
	Pistachios	
	Macadamias	
	Hazelnuts	

Grains: Below are the most common grain and seed choices. Legumes, beans, and nuts also provide a healthy amount of carbohydrates. Please check off the ones you will eat. Aim for whole grains first, not enriched whole wheat or bleached. These are acceptable whole grain foods and flours if including the bran, germ, and endosperm.

Amaranth	*Einkorn*	*Pasta*
Barley	*Ferro*	*Popped Corn*
Breads	*Flat Breads*	*Protein Bars*
Buckwheat	*Flour Tortillas*	*Quinoa*
Bulgar	*Forms of Whole Grains*	*Rice*
Cereal	*French Toast*	*Rice Tortillas*
Chips corn/flour/rice	*Graham Crackers*	*Rye*
Cookies - whole grain	*Granola*	*Seaweed Snacks*
Corn Tortillas	*Granola Bars*	*Spelt*
Corn/Popcorn	*Millet*	*Waffles*
Couscous	*Muffins*	*Wheat*
Crackers	*Oats/Oatmeal*	*Whole Grains*
Dried Fruit & Granola	*Pancakes*	*Wild Rice*

Seeds: Seeds have different nutrients for our bodies with some more power packed than others - there are hundreds of seeds to try.

MEAL PLANNING STEP 5: PUTTING IT TOGETHER – SIMPLY

It is time to see the fruits of your labor. I want to encourage you to use the Sample Blank Meal Plan pages and plug in all the preferred choices you just identified. If you are someone who just needs a plan, use any of the other meal plans provided on the following pages.

The following pages have these meal plans:

Sample Blank Meal Plans
Every Day Meal Plans
Gluten & Dairy Free Meal Plans
Gluten Free Meal Plans
Dairy Free Meal Plans
Lose Weight Meal Plans

Sample Blank Meal Plans

Use the Sample Blank Meal Plan charts: one meal plan for Monday, Wednesday, and Friday, and another meal plan for Tuesday, Thursday and the weekend).

If you have the same breakfast every day, you will most likely want to have different dinner choices. If you choose different breakfast choices most days of the week, you may find it acceptable to use the same 3-4 dinner ideas and just rotate. Which is easier for you to make? Go through each meal for one week by following these simple instructions:

1. Record the total calories goal you wish to meet every day at the top.
2. Record the selected calories from the Calorie Spreading Chart for each meal.
3. Vegetables: Choose at least 5 servings, up to 12 for each day, and write in your choices.
4. Fruit: Choose at least 2 to 4 fruits each day and write in your choices.
5. Protein: Aim for at least a little protein in every meal (10-25% of your daily intake).
6. Carbs: Remember you want between 45% and 65% of carbs during your day. With a 1,700 calorie diet, that is 765 to 1,105 calories of carbs.

If you need inspiration, plug-in options from the sample plans below.

3 Day Blank Meal Plan

Use this plan Monday, Wednesday, & Friday	
Total Daily Calories: _______	
Meal 1 Breakfast: _______ calories	
⇩Individual calories per food choice	
	Protein
	Carb/veggies
	(fruit)
Meal 2 Morning Snack: _______ calories	
	Protein, fruit, & or veggie
Meal 3 Lunch: _______ calories	
	Protein
	Vegetables
	Carb
	(fruit)
Meal 4 Afternoon Snack: _______ calories	
	(protein, fruit, or veggie)
Meal 5 Dinner: _______ calories	
	Protein
	Vegetables
	Carb
	(fruit)
Meal 6 Evening Snack: _______ calories	
	Protein
If your caloric needs are different, adjust this plan. Generally those who are starting out need a solid plan with higher calories, otherwise they binge eat on the weekends because they restricted so much during the week.	

Grill/cook extra meat on Monday to have it for the next couple of days.

4 Day Blank Meal Plan

Use this plan Tuesday, Thursday, and the Weekend	
Total Daily Calories: _______	
Meal 1 Breakfast: _______ calories	
⇩Individual calories per food choice	
	Protein
	Carb/veggies
	(fruit)
Meal 2 Morning Snack: _______ calories	
	Protein, fruit, & or veggie
Meal 3 Lunch: _______ calories	
	Protein
	Vegetables
	Carb
	(fruit)
Meal 4 Afternoon Snack: _______ calories	
	(protein, fruit, or veggie)
Meal 5 Dinner: _______ calories	
	Protein
	Vegetables
	Carb
	(fruit)
Meal 6 Evening Snack: _______ calories	
	Protein
If you caloric needs are different, adjust this plan. Generally those who are starting out need a solid plan with higher calories, otherwise they binge eat on the weekends because they restricted so much during the week.	

* Grill/cook extra meat on Monday to have it for the next couple of days.

Every Day Meal Plans

These two sample meal plans can be used every other day, and for as long as you would like. All recipes for the meal plans are in the section, Fit Recipes.

3 Day Meal Plan

Use this plan Monday, Wednesday, & Friday		
Total Daily Calories: 1750		
All recipes are in the Fit Recipes section of the Treasure Chest		
Breakfast — 400 calories		
400	Mon	½ c oatmeal, 1 TBS chia seeds, 1 c almond milk, ½ scoop vanilla protein powder, ½ banana
400	Wed	2 c high fiber cereal, 2 c almond milk, ¼ c blueberries
400	Fri	2 c high fiber cereal, 2 c almond milk, ¼ c blueberries or other berries
Snacks — 350 calories *Consume these throughout the day as needed*		
350	Mon	1 scoop protein powder, 1 c yogurt, ¼ c granola, ¼ c berries
350	Wed	½ scoop protein powder, apple, baby carrots, broccoli, 2 TB hummus
350	Fri	½ scoop protein powder, apple, baby carrots, broccoli, 2 TB hummus
Lunch — 500 calories		
500	Mon	Power Salad, 1 c almond milk, 1 c cottage cheese, ½ banana
500	Wed	Tuna Pouch, 4-5 melba toast, spinach, onion, tomatoes, 1 c almond milk
500	Fri	Left over chicken breast, tortilla, salsa, blk beans, onions, avocado, spinach
Dinner — 500 calories		
500	Mon	Hidden Spaghetti, 3 whole grain crackers, 2 c almond milk
500	Wed	Chicken Breast Salsa Crock Pot, blk beans, onions, chips, ¼ avocado
500	Fri	Corn shell tacos/tortillas, (chix, beef, fish) salsa, blk beans, onions, chips, ¼ avocado
If your caloric needs are different, adjust this plan. Generally those who are starting out need a solid plan with higher calories, otherwise they binge eat on the weekends because they restricted so much during the week.		

* Grill/cook extra meat to have it for the next couple of days.

4 Day Meal Plan

Use this plan Tuesday, Thursday, & Weekends		
Total Daily Calories: 1750		
All recipes are in the Fit Recipes section of the Treasure Chest		
Breakfast — 400 calories		
400	**Tues**	Omelet (prepped veggies from Monday's salad), steamed broccoli, ½ grapefruit, 1 c almond milk
400	**Thurs**	Protein smoothie
400	**Sat**	2 hard boiled eggs, 2 slices bacon, ½ lg banana, 2 c almond milk
400	**Sun**	1-2-3 Pancakes, 2 c coconut or almond milk
Snacks — 350 calories *Consume these throughout the day as needed*		
350	**Tues**	20 almonds, 2 celery, baby carrots, 2 TBS hummus, green tea
350	**Thurs**	½ scoop protein powder, hard boiled egg, broccoli, cauliflower, hummus
350	**Sat**	Omelet (prepped veggies from Fri dinner)
350	**Sun**	20 almonds, 2 celery, baby carrots, 2 TBS hummus, green tea
Lunch — 500 calories		
500	**Tues**	Left-over Hidden Spaghetti and ½ grapefruit
500	**Thurs**	Tuna Pouch, 4-5 melba toast, spinach, onion, tomatoes, 1 c almond milk
500	**Sat**	Mexican Power Salad (prepped from night prior), 1 c almond milk, 1 c cottage cheese, ½ lg banana
500	**Sun**	100% Turkey/Beef hotdog on grill, 7 chips, salsa, Power Salad
Dinner — 500 calories		
500	**Tues**	Grilled/broiled tilapia or fish on Power Salad, ½ c quinoa, 2 c coconut or almond milk
500	**Thurs**	Grilled chicken breast, sweet potato, ¼ c zucchini with pinch of cheese, iced green tea with lemon
500	**Sat**	Repeat meal or go out for date night
500	**Sun**	Crock Pot BBQ Chicken, ½ c quinoa or rice, pickles, celery, 2 TBS hummus

* Grill/cook extra meat on Monday to have it for the next couple of days.

Gluten & Dairy Free Meal Plans

The following four meal plans are gluten and/or dairy free. Read the recommendations at the top of each plan. Your calorie necessity may be more or less than the recommended serving size. Add to or subtract from your serving size as needed. In my meals that consist of lean protein such as fish or chicken, I often sauté my vegetables with sliced tomatoes, onions, garlic, cayenne pepper, turmeric, and basil to make them pop with flavor.

Gluten & Dairy Free Meal Plan

Use this plan Monday, Wednesday, & Friday	
Use this as a guide for your caloric intake. Your calories may need to change based off your activity and dietary needs. These below calories listed are general and may be higher or lower based on your brand names.	
Estimated Caloric Total: 1670 calories	
Meal 1 Breakfast — 320 calories	
320	Smoothie: 10oz. almond or coconut milk, ½ cup spinach or kale, 1 scoop protein powder, banana, ¼ cup strawberries
Meal 2 Morning Snack — 90 calories	
90	1 cup fresh carrots with light ranch **(40cals)**
Meal 3 Lunch — 460 calories	
90	3oz. pouch packed tuna, sea salt and ½ TBS light ranch
200	Protein bar (with 5g or less of added sugar)
70	1 cup broccoli **(30cals)**, 1 TBS light ranch **(40cals)**, or 1 TBS hummus **(30cals)**
100	Banana
Meal 4 Afternoon Snack — 105 calories	
105	15 almonds or walnuts
Meal 5 Dinner — 620 calories	
200	Turkey, beef, or chicken cooked in coconut oil with herbs and any spices*
200	Fresh loaded veggie salad with ½ avocado
220	Quinoa **(220cals)**, or sweet potato with 1 TBS organic grass-fed butter and sea salt **(230cals)**
Meal 6 PM Snack — 75 calories	
75	Hard boiled egg or protein drink
If your caloric needs are different, adjust this plan. Generally those who are starting out need a solid plan with higher calories, otherwise they binge eat on the weekends because they restricted so much during the week.	

* Grill/cook extra meat on Monday to have it for the next couple of days.

Gluten & Dairy Free Meal Plan

Use this plan Tuesday, Thursday, & Saturday (Sunday you choose)

30-45 minutes before exercise, try ½ a protein drink. Then when done, drink the rest. Don't forget to add this to your total calories.

Estimated Caloric Total: 1620-1650 calories

Meal 1 Breakfast — 265-295 calories

265 Option 1 — 1 cup cold cereal, 1 cup almond or coconut milk **(180cals)**, and 1 cup berries **(85cals)**

295 Option 2 —omelet: 2 eggs, onions, spinach, peppers, mushrooms **(210cals)** and 1 cup berries **(85cals)**

Meal 2 Lunch — 480 calories

180 Small salad with as many veggies as you can put on it, 2 TBS light ranch

200 Deli meat wrap - brown rice tortilla **(130cals)**, 3 turkey slices **(35cals)**, spinach, cucumbers, peppers, onions

100 Small peach or pear

Meal 3 Afternoon Snack — 200 calories

200 Protein bar (with 5g or less of added sugar and at least 5g of fiber)

Meal 4 Dinner — 595 calories

140 Chicken breast or your choice of meat with fresh garlic, lemon juice, and fresh basil (put raw meat in crock pot for easy cooking)

215 1 cup brown rice **(215cals) or** Gluten-free: sweet potato with bacon bits and 1 TBS organic butter **(240cals)**

75 2 servings of veggies: green beans, carrots, or corn on cob

Meal 5: PM Snack — 80 calories

80 Apple

* If you need something extra, try taking a cheat meal and not an entire cheat day.

Gluten Free Meal Plans

These next two meal plans are gluten free and are to be used every other day and for as long as you would like.

Gluten Free Meal Plan

Use this plan Monday, Wednesday, & Friday	
Use this as a guide for your caloric intake. Your calories may need to change based off your activity and dietary needs. These below calories listed are general and may be higher or lower based on your brand names.	
Estimated Caloric Total: 1660 calories	
Meal 1 Breakfast — 435 Calories	
295	2 egg omelet with mushrooms, onions, zucchini, tomatoes, greens
30	1 cup of steamed broccoli
100	Banana
Meal 2 Morning Snack — 170 calories	
85	1 cup Fresh berries
85	½ cup Greek plain yogurt
Meal 3 Lunch — 435 calories	
90	3oz. pouch packed tuna, sea salt and 1 TBS light ranch
215	Brown rice tortilla, spinach, onions
50	1 cup baby carrots
80	Apple
Meal 4 Afternoon Snack — 105 calories	
105	15 almonds or walnuts
Meal 5 Dinner — 585 calories	
200	Turkey, beef, or chicken cooked in coconut oil with herbs and spices*
200	Fresh loaded veggie salad with ½ avocado
220	1 cup quinoa
Meal 6 PM Snack: 80 calories	
80	Cottage cheese or hard boiled egg

* Grill/cook extra meat on Monday to have it for the next couple of days.

Gluten Free Meal Plan

Tuesday, Thursday, & Saturday

30-45 minutes before exercise, try ½ a protein drink. Then when done, drink the rest. Don't forget to add this to your total calories.

Use this plan Tuesday, Thursday, & Saturday (Sunday you choose)

Meal 1: Breakfast — 320-410 calories

320 Option 1 — 10oz. smoothie: almond, coconut, or milk with ½ cup spinach or kale, 1 scoop vanilla protein powder, banana, ¼ cup strawberries

410 Option 2 — 10oz. smoothie: almond, coconut, or milk with ½ cup kale, 1 scoop chocolate protein power, 1 TBS cocoa powder, 1 TBS peanut butter

Meal 2: Lunch — 635 calories

350 5oz. cooked chicken breast strips

200 2 cups salad; broccoli, spinach, zucchini, mushrooms, onions, zucchini, tomatoes, dried fruit, green and red peppers

40 ½ cup skim cottage cheese

45 1 cup watermelon or cantaloupe

Meal 3: Afternoon Snack — 100

1 cup yogurt

Meal 4: Dinner — 600 calories

120 3oz. Tilapia with Italian seasoning, or other seasoning

200 Fresh loaded veggie salad with ½ avocado

280 Baked potato, light sour cream, real bacon bits, chives (onions)

Estimated Total: 1655-1745

* Grill/cook extra meat on Monday to have it for the next couple of days.

Dairy Free Meal Plans

These next two meal plans are dairy free and are to be used weekly every other day.

Dairy Free Meal Plan

Use this plan Monday, Wednesday, & Friday	
Depending on when you choose to exercise, 30-45 minutes beforehand drink protein drink and eat the next meal within 30-45 minutes after your workout.	
Estimated Caloric Total: 1670 Calories	
Meal 1 Breakfast — 355 calories	
295	2 egg omelet with mushrooms, onions, zucchini, tomatoes, greens
30	1 cup of steamed broccoli
Meal 2 Lunch — 480 calories	
180	Small salad with as many veggies as you can put on it, 2 TBS light ranch
200	Deli meat wrap - brown rice tortilla **(130cals)**, 3 turkey slices **(35cals)**, spinach, cucumbers, peppers, onions
100	Small peach, banana, or pear
Meal 3 Afternoon Snack — 200 calories	
200	Protein bar (with 5g or less of added sugar and at least 5g of fiber)
Meal 4 Dinner — 585 calories	
300	Tuna, tilapia, salmon, fish
200	2 cups favorite vegetables
85	1 cup fresh berries or dried fruit
Meal 5 PM Snack — 50 calories	
50	1 small scoop protein drink
* If you need something extra, try taking a cheat meal and not an entire cheat day.	

Dairy Free Meal Plan

Use this plan Tuesday, Thursday, & Saturday (Sunday you choose)

30-45 minutes before exercise, try ½ a protein drink. Then when done, drink the rest. Don't forget to add this to your total calories.

Estimated Total: 1680 calories

Meal 1: Breakfast — 355 calories

½ cup oatmeal **(150cals)**, ¼ scoop protein powder **(30cals)**, 1 tsp cinnamon, ¼ cup raisins **(130cals)**, 3 walnuts **(45cals)**

Meal 2:Lunch — 480 calories

380 Large salad with as many veggies as you can put on it, 2 TBS light ranch, hard boiled egg, real bacon bits, dried fruit

100 Small peach, banana, or pear

Meal 3: Afternoon Snack — 200 calories

Protein bar (with 5g or less of added sugar and at least 5g of fiber)

Meal 4: Dinner — 595 calories

150 3oz. Chicken breast or your choice of meat with fresh garlic, lemon juice, and fresh basil (put raw meat in crock pot for easy cooking)

215 1 cup Brown rice **(215cals)**

75 2 servings of veggies: green beans, carrots, or corn on cob

Meal 5: PM Snack — 50 calories

1 small scoop protein drink

* If you need something extra, try taking a cheat meal and not an entire cheat day.

Lose Weight Meal Plans

The following meal plans target weight loss. To be used every other day. You can use this meal plan as long as you would like.

Lose Weight Meal Plan

Use this plan Monday, Wednesday, & Friday
Use this as a guide for your caloric intake. Your calories may need to change based off your activity and dietary needs. These below calories listed are general and may be higher or lower based on your brand names.
Estimated Caloric Total: 1395 calories
Meal 1 Breakfast — 320 calories
240 3 egg omelet with onions, peppers, tomatoes, basil, mushrooms, garlic
80 Banana
0 Green tea with ½ lemon
Meal 2 Morning Snack — 110 calories
60 2 stalks celery and 1 cup carrots
55 2 TBS humus
Meal 3 Lunch — 355 calories
90 3oz. tuna pouch
215 1 cup brown rice
50 1 cup steamed broccoli
Meal 4 Afternoon Snack — 150 calories
80 Apple, pear, peach or favorite fruit
70 10 almonds
Meal 5 Dinner — 460 calories
150 1 cup Greek yogurt (plain or under 11g sugar)
230 ½ cup naked granola (under 7g sugar)
80 1 cup blueberries
* Grill/cook extra meat on Monday to have it for the next couple of days.

Lose Weight Meal Plan

Use this plan Tuesday, Thursday, & the Weekend	
30-45 minutes before exercise, try ½ a protein drink. Then when done, drink the rest. Don't forget to add this to your total calories.	
Estimated Total: 1320 calories	
Meal 1 Breakfast — 260 calories	
180	½ cup oatmeal **(150cals)**, ¼ scoop protein powder **(30cals)**, 1 tsp cinnamon
80	½ cup of fresh strawberries or kiwi
0	Green tea with ½ lemon
Meal 2 Morning Snack — 170 calories	
70	3 eggs whites omelet with onions, spinach, mushrooms, green pepper ½ avocado
100	1 cup of either carrots, black beans, green beans, or broccoli
Meal 3 Dinner — 400 calories	
350	5oz. cooked chicken breast
50	½ cup broccoli and ½ cup green beans
Meal 4 Afternoon Snack — 80 calories	
	Apple
Meal 5 Dinner — 410 calories	
150	Tilapia or salmon cooked in coconut oil with spices
260	Fresh salad with veggies, ½ cup cottage cheese, and 5 almonds, hard boiled egg, ½ avocado
* Grill/cook extra meat on Monday to have it for the next couple of days.	

Quick Tips on When to Eat

Pre-Workout

1. Split your full regular meal in half—eat half now and half after exercise.
2. Try a smaller snack: protein bar, hard boiled egg, a glass of milk, or fruit.
3. Fuel your body throughout the entire day, so you have enough fuel when you perform an evening workout.
4. Consume a smaller portion at least 30-45 minutes before exercise.
    a. protein bar
    b. yogurt
    c. banana
    d. liquid protein drink
    e. small bowl of cereal/oatmeal
    f. nuts or seeds

During Workout

1. While performing cardio exercise, aim to drink about 3 ounces of water every 20 minutes.
2. Once you hit an hour of hard training, such as running, consume some type of liquid food if you are going to continue exercising—something light with sugar such as a sports drink or fruit.

Post Workout

1. Consume liquid protein after weight lifting within 15-30 minutes. If it's not quite time for one of your main meals, enjoy a healthy snack.
2. If you exercise in the evening, it is perfectly fine and encouraged to eat something before bed, focus on protein.
    a. Protein drink
    b. Hard boiled egg
    c. Cottage cheese

FIT RECIPES

Fit Breakfasts

1-2-3 Pre-workout Pancakes

INGREDIENTS: ½ cup oats, ½ cup fat-free cottage cheese, 2 egg whites, ½ tsp. cinnamon, ½ tsp. vanilla extract, 1 tbsp. flavored protein powder

DIRECTIONS: Mix all the ingredients together in a blender until it resembles pancake batter. Pour into a non-stick skillet and cook for 2-3 minutes on each side. Top with fresh fruit.

Fit Toast

INGREDIENTS: 1 scoop flavored protein powder, 2 slices of whole grain bread (or Ezekiel Bread), ½ cup egg whites, ¼ cup milk, 1 banana, cinnamon

DIRECTIONS: Mix egg whites, milk, and protein powder together in a small bowl. Add cinnamon to taste. Dip the slices of bread into the mixture. Place the batter-covered bread on a non-stick skillet and cook for 2-3 minutes on each side, then remove from heat. Cut the banana into small pieces and sprinkle on top of bread. Add fruit or a little Cool Whip for taste.

Power Protein Muffins

INGREDIENTS: 3 large eggs, 3 tbsp. oil, ¼ cup half and half, 5 scoops vanilla or chocolate protein powder, 2 tsp. baking powder, ¼ cup brown sugar (or stevia), 1 cup blueberries, ½ cup fat-free cream cheese, ¼ tsp. cinnamon

DIRECTIONS: Preheat oven to 375 F. Line 9 muffin tins with cups and non-stick spray. Mix cream cheese and cinnamon in a small bowl. Mix eggs, oil, and half and half, then protein powder, baking power and sugar (or sweetener), stirring thoroughly. Combine berries. Pour into the muffin tins. Bake for 15-20 minutes or until muffins begin to brown at the top.

Vegan Oatmeal Banana Waffles

INGREDIENTS: 2 cups oatmeal, 1 ripe banana, 2 cups water (or almond milk), 1 tsp. vanilla, sprinkle to a tsp. baking powder

DIRECTIONS: Blend oats, banana, and water (or Almond milk) in a food processor. Gradually add the vanilla and baking soda. Once the mixture is blended, leave it for five minutes to set. Pour into your waffle maker—they take about 5-8 minutes to cook.

Cinnamon Protein Apples

INGREDIENTS: 3 large Fuji apples, 1 tbsp. cinnamon, vanilla protein powder

DIRECTIONS: Slice apples and place them into a sealed plastic bag. Pour cinnamon and protein powder into the bag. Shake vigorously, plate and serve.

Omelets

INGREDIENTS: 2-3 large eggs (I use 2 eggs and 1 egg white), onion, peppers, mushrooms

DIRECTIONS: Chop veggies and toss in preferred oil. Allow to cook for 1-2 minutes and then pour in eggs. Cook. Serve with salsa or fresh avocado.

Fit Lunches

Protein Smoothies

**Sometimes smoothies can be thick if the fruit was previously frozen. Use less ice or use more milk for your desired consistency. These below yield a 16-ounce smoothie.*

Strawberry Banana Smoothie

10 oz. Unsweetened vanilla almond milk, ½ fresh or frozen banana, 2 frozen or fresh strawberries, protein powder, 8 ice cubes

Mocha Java Smoothie

10 oz. unsweetened vanilla almond milk, chocolate protein powder, 1 tbsp. instant coffee or 1-2 tbsp. organic coffee/espresso, 10 ice cubes

Low Calorie Super Smoothie

10 oz. unsweetened vanilla almond milk, 1 tbsp. milled chia seeds, handful of kale or spinach, 1 tbsp. milled flaxseed, ¼ cup mixed frozen berries, protein powder, 10 ice cubes

Chocolate Banana & Oats Smoothie

10 oz. unsweetened vanilla almond milk, 1 fresh or frozen banana, ½ cup rolled oats, 1 tbsp, cocoa powder, chocolate or vanilla protein powder, 6-8 ice cubes

Fiber Filled Tortilla

INGREDIENTS: Whole grain tortilla (high fiber), 1 cup organic spinach, 3 tbsp. organic onions, ¼ mashed avocado, ¼ cup low sodium black beans, 2 tbsp. organic tomatoes, 3 tbsp. fresh salsa

DIRECTIONS: Place ingredients on tortilla and warm or enjoy temperature as is. Option to add chicken, tuna, beef, lamb, cucumbers, squash, olives, diced carrots, diced celery, diced peppers, diced mushrooms, low fat cheese. Serve with ½ cup plain Greek yogurt, ¼ cup blueberries, and a glass of almond milk.

Power Parfait

INGREDIENTS: ½ cup low-fat plain Greek yogurt, ¼ cup frozen or fresh blueberries or mixed berries, 10 almonds, ¼ cup rolled oats or low sugar granola, 1 tbsp. organic chia seeds

DIRECTIONS: Layer as listed. Enjoy with a glass of almond milk.

Power 10 Salad

INGREDIENTS: 2 cups organic spinach, kale, strips of cabbage or leafy greens and 9 other ingredients of your choice: cubed beets, bell peppers, radishes, tomatoes, any type onions, carrots, sweet corn, broccoli, celery, cucumber, snow peas, sugar snap peas, zucchini, black olives, cauliflower, mushrooms, sliced almonds, sliced walnuts, any type of desired seeds, cranberries, raisins, low calorie croutons, diced or strips of cooked meat—chicken, shrimp, turkey, ham or steak

DIRECTIONS: Layer as desired. Enjoy with low sodium cottage cheese or low sugar yogurt as the dressing, or a light dressing.

Fit Dinners

Chicken Breast Salsa Crock Pot

INGREDIENTS: frozen chicken breasts (any desired amount),12 oz. jar of salsa

DIRECTIONS: Place frozen chicken breasts in crock pot. Pour a bottle of salsa (fresh salsa is better) over the chicken. Cover. Turn on low for 5-8 hours or high for 3-5 hours depending on the amount of chicken and crock pot temps. *Eat this plain, with rice, or inside whole grain tortillas with black beans, onions, and guacamole. You can use the next day in soups, sandwiches, or casseroles.

Crock Pot BBQ Chicken

INGREDIENTS: frozen chicken breasts (any desired amount), 1 bottle of low sugar BBQ sauce (I use Cookies brand with 7 grams of sugar.)

DIRECTIONS: Place frozen chicken breasts in crock pot. Pour a bottle of BBQ sauce over the chicken. Cover. Turn on low for 5-8 hours or high for 3-5 hours depending on the amount of chicken and crock pot temps.

Crock Pot Taco Soup

INGREDIENTS: 1 lb. raw grass fed organic beef, 1 taco seasoning packet, 1 can or fresh organic diced tomatoes, 1 can low sodium or soaked black beans, 1 can or fresh organic corn, 1 cup fresh salsa, 1 diced onion

DIRECTIONS: Combine all ingredients in order in the crock pot. Add a little water to desired consistency (usually 1 cup). Cover and cook on low for 5+ hours (depending on the crock pot). Stir and mix well before serving. Yields 6 servings.

Fit Quinoa

INGREDIENTS: 1 cup quinoa, 2 cups water, 1 tsp. each of salt and paprika, 2 tbsp. vinegar, 1 tsp. each of dried thyme and rosemary, 1 tsp. garlic, juice of half a lime (optional), 2 cups chopped spinach leaves, ½ cup chopped green onion, 1 cup chopped sun-dried tomatoes, ¼ cup cubed feta cheese, ¼ cup whole black olives, 1 cup cubed roasted pumpkin or squash, a dash of olive oil

DIRECTIONS: Bring water, salt, paprika, thyme, rosemary, and garlic to a boil in a large saucepan. Boil quinoa like rice (or follow directions on quinoa package). Add vinegar. Stir. Add lime juice, olive oil, pumpkin/squash, sun-dried tomatoes, olives, feta cheese, spinach and green onions. Toss and mix gently. Enjoy with an apple and unsweetened lemon iced tea.

Grilled/Baked Tilapia

INGREDIENTS: 1 pound tilapia fillets, or desired amount, 1 lemon or lime, and spice mixture with a ½ teaspoon of each: paprika, oregano, garlic powder, cumin, cayenne pepper

GRILLED DIRECTIONS: Preheat grill. Lightly coat a piece of tin foil with oil, sprinkle ½ spice mixture on foil, add fillets and remaining spice mixture. Wrap foil and grill over low-medium heat until fish flakes with fork. About 4 minutes per side to grill. Enjoy with grilled veggies.

BAKED DIRECTIONS: Preheat oven to 450 F. Line 9x13 pan with foil. Lightly coat tin foil with oil, sprinkle ½ spice mixture on foil, add fillets and remaining spice mixture. Bake for 10 minutes or until fish flakes with fork. Serve with steamed veggies.

Hidden Spaghetti

INGREDIENTS: 1 jar organic pasta sauce (store bought optional), as many veggies as you can find (spinach, onions, zucchini, squash, carrots, mushrooms, green and red peppers, tomatoes, etc), ground beef or ground sausage

DIRECTIONS: This is your opportunity to make your spaghetti pop. Prepare as normal (using organic spaghetti sauce if you can) and add as many veggies as possible. Some ingredients I usually add and "hide" in this Hidden Spaghetti are shredded carrots, shredded zucchini, onions, and mushrooms. You may need to add more spaghetti sauce. Serve over rice or whole grain noodles.

Mexican Power Salad

INGREDIENTS: A power salad has at least 10 ingredients such as: corn, black beans, onions, rice, lettuce, salsa, guacamole, and Mexican items.

Loaded Sweet Potato

INGREDIENTS: 1 large sweet potato, 2 tbsp. plain Greek yogurt, 3 tbsp. salsa, ½ cup low sodium black beans, 1 stalk diced green onion, dash chili powder, dash cumin, dash paprika, pinch of salt or 1 tsp. taco seasoning (optional: 2 tbsp. mozzarella, 1 strip of bacon, 1 tbsp. low-fat sour cream, 1 tbsp. organic butter, 1 tsp. fresh cilantro)

DIRECTIONS: Preheat oven to 400 F (or use microwave for a super quick meal—I do not suggest doing it often, but when in a time crunch this is an option). Wash potato, poke a few fork holes in it and bake 45 minutes (microwave for 8-10 minutes). Add taco seasoning mix or other spices to Greek yogurt. Stir well. Top sweet potato with drained beans, salsa, and the yogurt mixture. Add any optional items and enjoy!

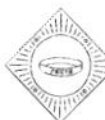

Low Calorie Power Spaghetti

INGREDIENTS: 1 lb grass fed ground beef, handful baby carrots, 1 zucchini, 1 onion, 1 cup spinach, 1-15 oz. can tomato sauce, 1 can diced tomato, 1 tsp. garlic, pinch of salt, 1 tbsp. fresh oregano or Italian seasoning, 1 spaghetti squash

DIRECTIONS: Split spaghetti squash in half and carve out seeds and stem. Place ½ cup of water on the inside of one half, place other half on top to close it. Place squash in microwave safe dish for 10 minutes. Cook beef, drain any grease, add tomato sauce and spices. Use the food processor to chop veggies slightly. Pour chopped ingredients, including diced tomato, into sauce. Mix well. Take out squash and carefully open halves. Use a fork to carve out the strands of squash—it will resemble spaghetti noodles. Serve with sauce.

Whole Grain Tuna Melt

INGREDIENTS: uncooked 10 oz. box whole grain noodles, large can/fresh cooked tuna, 1 cup low fat shredded cheese

DIRECTIONS: Combine all ingredients together in a mixing bowl and spread in 9x13 greased pan. Bake at 350 F for 20 minutes. Yields 6 servings.

Snappy Side Dishes

Cauliflower Fried Rice

INGREDIENTS: 1 head of cauliflower, 1 tbsp. extra-virgin olive oil, 2 garlic cloves, 2 stalks green onion, salt and pepper to taste, 1 lime, ¼ cup chopped fresh cilantro

DIRECTIONS: Discard core of cauliflower and dry completely. Coarsely chop into florets, and then place in food processor and pulse (do not over process as it will become mushy–it should resemble rice). On medium heat add olive oil, garlic and green onions. Sauté, increase heat slightly, and add cauliflower. Cover and cook for 5-6 minutes frequently stirring until it is slightly crispy. Top with a squeeze of lime and chopped cilantro. Enjoy with your favorite main dish.

Steamed Broccoli

INGREDIENTS: fresh broccoli

DIRECTIONS: Place 2-4 serving sizes of broccoli in a microwave-safe bowl with ¼ cup water, cover with paper towel, and cook for 2 minutes. You can always steam these on the stove!

Steamed Micro Sweet Corn

INGREDIENTS: sweet corn

DIRECTIONS: Pop your sweet corn on the cob, still wrapped in the husk, in the microwave for 10 minutes. When you take it out, unwrap, and the silk will fall right off. Cut it or eat it right off the cob. *Microwaves have been considered to lessen the quality of your food. The research is still out to adequately indicate otherwise. If you need a quick vegetable on your plate and do not have much time, in my opinion, it is better you use it than not serve a vegetable.

Healthy Desserts

EASY Homemade Oatmeal Options The below four recipes have some fun options. Add other ingredients to make these foods pop, such as different flavors of protein powder, ¼ cup chia seeds, 1 tbsp. mini chocolate chips or peanuts, chunks of apple, cocoa powder, and milled flaxseed.

Oatmeal Banana Biscuits:

INGREDIENTS: 1 cup oatmeal, 1 banana

DIRECTIONS: Mash together and shape into biscuits. Bake at 350 F for 10 minutes.

Oatmeal Applesauce Biscuits:

INGREDIENTS: 1 cup oatmeal, 1 cup applesauce

DIRECTIONS: Mix and shape like cookies. Bake at 350 F for 15 minutes.

Protein Bars:

INGREDIENTS: 2 cups oatmeal, 1 cup protein powder, 1 cup milled flax, 1 cup peanut butter, and 1/8 cup honey

DIRECTIONS: Melt peanut butter and honey to a liquid. Add other ingredients. Mix with hands or wooden spoon. Spread in an 8x8 pan.

Cookie Dough Dip:

INGREDIENTS: 1 can chickpeas drained/rinsed, ¼ cup milk, ¼ cup almond butter, 1/8 tsp. salt.

DIRECTIONS: Place in a blender for a few seconds until creamy. Eat with flat pretzels or veggie sticks. (Optional ingredients: 2-3 packets stevia, chocolate chips.)

Chia Pudding

INGREDIENTS: ½ cup almond or coconut milk, 2 tbsp. chia seeds, 1 tbsp. honey or real maple syrup (optional: ¼ tsp. cinnamon, ¼ tsp. Nutmeg, dash of stevia)

DIRECTIONS: Mix all ingredients together in a small bowl and cover. Place in fridge for 10 minutes and up to 4 days.

Avocado Cookies

INGREDIENTS: 1 soft avocado, 1 banana, ¼ cup cocoa powder

DIRECTIONS: Mash all ingredients using a blender or food processor or by hand. Add optional ingredients of 1 tsp. vanilla, stevia, 1 tbsp. honey, or mini chocolate chips if you want it sweeter. Cook at 350 F for 10 or so minutes. Do not feel bad if you eat the whole batch—they are delicious! Eat right away or place in fridge in airtight container.

Simple Snack List

There are so many different types of snack choices, and they will always be revolving due to our food supply, but here are a few easy choices.

Simple Anytime Food Choices

- Eggs—any way you like them, plus it is the cheapest and healthiest snack around
- Veggies—carrots, celery, bell peppers, broccoli, with hummus, peanut butter, or yogurt
- Fruit
- Bowl of whole grain cereal, add fruit
- Salad—if your greens are prepped, it is easy to grab it and go
- Popcorn—low salt (try seasonings on it)
- Trail mix or nuts—almonds, peanuts, walnuts or seeds in general
- Dairy—cottage cheese, string cheese, milk, or plain yogurt
- 1 Hard boiled egg drizzled with olive oil and sprinkled with freshly ground black pepper
- Part-skim mozzarella cheese stick
- 2 Tablespoons peanut butter (pair with sliced apples)
- 8-ounce Glass of milk (pair with any snack or indulge with two small cookies)
- Shredded cheddar (melt on 10 whole grain tortilla chips in microwave)
- 1 Slice Swiss cheese (pair with a handful of grapes)
- 2 Slices natural deli turkey (roll with lettuce and Dijon mustard)
- 6-ounce Cup of yogurt (blend with fruit and milk for a frosty smoothie)
- Greek yogurt (topped with frozen raspberries and blackberries)

10 Grams of Protein or More

- 6-ounce Cup low-fat flavored Greek yogurt
- 1/3 Cup tuna with whole grain crackers
- ½ Cup cottage cheese with sliced pears
- 1-ounce Diced canned chicken breast tossed with light mayo and hot sauce with celery
- 12-ounce Non-fat latte

Portable Protein Snacks

- Mix plain Greek yogurt with flavored protein powder
- Combine cheese slices with apple slices

- Top off your cottage cheese with berries
- Low sodium and natural beef or turkey jerky
- Hard boiled egg
- Trail mix of seeds and almonds
- Low sodium lunch meat wrapped around string cheese
- Dip celery in natural peanut butter and top it off with raisins
- Mix whey protein with almond milk and yogurt
- Spread peanut butter on a brown rice cake with banana
- Mix salsa in your cottage cheese

DINNER PLANNING TIPS

1. **Keep It Simple**
   When in a hurry, meal planning is pushed aside because we know we can grab just about anything on the go through drive-thru or by making a simple phone call. The issue is the *types* of fast choices we are making. Eating at home can be easy. Do not feel like you need to do something NEW every week! Rotate through a generic schedule. Like this below:

Crock pot **Mondays,** Taco **Tuesdays,** Whatever **Wednesdays,** Leftover **Thursdays,** Out to eat **Fridays,** Order-in **Saturdays,** Family Meal **Sundays**

Mexican **Mondays,** Italian **Tuesdays,** American **Wednesdays,** Greek **Thursdays,** French **Fridays,** Left Over **Saturdays,** Eat Out **Sundays**

2. **Decide What Type of Night It Will Be**

Make Your Own	Outside	Got Time to Prepare
Potato bar Tacos Salad	Grill Picnic Open fire	Crock pot Bake night prior
Breakfast For Dinner	Take Turns Dinner	Got No Time to Prep
Scrambled eggs Omelets Breakfast casserole	Kids make dinner Spouse makes dinner Family makes dinner	Crock pot Store bought prepped

3. **Write It Down**
   Simply write down what a simple week could look like for your dinners, then KEEP that paper and use it next week or the week after. After two or three weeks of this, you have yourself a plan that works for you and your family.

 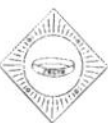

4. **Dinner Ideas**

Below is a list of healthier go-to dinner options. These are the choices I use the most, and they are relatively easy, quick, and healthy. There is no grilled cheese or mac-and-cheese, in fact there is not much cheese at all. You can always add whatever your family chooses to make it work for you. Once you master the recipes, reference this chart for quick meal ideas!

On the Grill	**Baked (night prior?)**	**Crock Pot Meals**
Burgers	Chicken (with dressing)	Pulled Chicken
Hotdogs	Chicken & Seasonings	Pulled Beef
Sausage Links	Tilapia	Roast & Veggies
Shish-k-bobs	Salmon	Spaghetti & Meatballs
Chicken	Steak (flank, peppered)	Meatball Subs
Tofu	Chicken Strips	Spaghetti Sauce
Fish	Chicken & Pasta	Chili Dogs
Steaks	Meatloaf	Lasagna
Vegetables	Teriyaki Chicken	Chicken, Beef Enchilada
	Chicken (ginger, honey,	Italian P Roast
Use Grilled Meat & Make:	parmesan, salsa)	Salsa Chicken
Sliders	Stuffed Shells	Chicken Fajitas
Tacos	Veggie Pizza	
Enchiladas	Spaghetti	**Sandwiches & Wraps**
Quesadillas	Mexican Lasagna	Any type of wraps
Wraps		Chicken-Strip Wraps
Sandwiches	**Stove Top & Skillet**	Bacon, Lettuce & Tomato
Fajitas	Rice (pilaf, seasoned)	Sloppy Joes
	Jambalaya	Reuben
Soups	Rice, Beans & Beef	Chicken Salad
Black Bean Soup	Red Beans & Rice	Tuna Salad
Split Pea Soup	Spaghetti (beef, chicken)	Use: bread, pita, wrap
Vegetable		
Potato Soup	**Salads**	**Quick & Fast**
Beef Stew	Taco Salad	Cold Cereal
Taco Soup	Fruit Salad	Sandwiches
Chicken Noodle	Egg Salad	Baked Potato Bar
Chicken & Dumplings	Tuna Salad	Omelets
Goulash	Spinach Salad	Yogurt & Granola

ACKNOWLEDGMENTS

To my husband, thank you for literally providing and paving the path for this journey as we raised our six children side by side. I am beyond blessed God crossed our paths that one day during cheerleading practice in college. Who knew 20 years into marriage we'd have all these teenagers? I love you with all my heart. You make my heart full with love and laughter.

Thank you to my children—Grant, Grace, Glory, Hope, Harmony, and Mercie—for showing me that I am not a perfect mom, and that I don't have to be. I pray you will fulfill God's perfect plan He has for each of you. I am thrilled God chose me to be your mom. I love you all so dearly—you all make my heart smile.

Thank you Mom, for training me and raising me in the Scriptures, always being an amazing role model, giving me sound wisdom, letting me make mistakes and allowing me to learn from them, and for being there even though I was not always there for you. You are beyond a true Proverbs 31 woman and I am one of the most blessed women in the world to have you as my mother.

Thank you, Dr. Marianna VonMuenster, for being that wise friend who always knows what to say when I need to hear it. Conversations are as easy as eating chips and salsa with you. I am forever grateful our husbands are besties too. Thank you for praying for me, encouraging me, and making me laugh constantly!

To Tracy Dunn, my sidewalk friend (the lady I ran after on the street one early morning) who God placed in my path about five years later to help edit this book. Thank you for not thinking I was a crazy woman on the sidewalk, and for writing your follow up article on our encounter. You lend much wisdom and I am richer for knowing you. Thank you!

Thank you Laura Kuster for answering God's call! You are the one I prayed for in the quiet of my bedroom. A few days later, you came to me telling me God was directing you to help edit my book. From the grassroots of organizing to the dedication of my first edits, you were a gifted and tremendous help.

Erin Engelbrecht, thank you for being that first woman to tell me I was good enough and should print and publish this. Your encouragement was exactly what God had placed in my path. You are an amazing mother and role model and I am so blessed to have you in my life and as a part of my wise counsel.

To Elisa Green, thank you for always being up for a walk. We are those non-stop talking friends. We somehow conquer the world on our walks and talks and it refreshes me to spend time with you. Thank you for giving me wise counsel. You are a true friend.

My Pilot Group, what an amazing group of ladies you are! Thank you for taking the time to do this for me. I pray blessings for you and your personal journeys.

Shawn Reimers, thanks for the blessings of your time with photography. You are gifted and I pray blessings on your future endeavors.

ABOUT THE AUTHOR

Sarah Hansel was raised in Florida and studied in Oklahoma where she met her husband—on their collegiate cheerleading team. After she graduated from Oral Roberts University with her bachelor's, her increased love of health and fitness led her to over a dozen different certification specialties in personal training, group fitness instruction, nutrition, and wellness coaching. She actively teaches various fitness classes weekly and enjoys speaking and teaching practical health and wellness to individuals and businesses, nationally and internationally. Sarah and her husband have six children, which gives them one busy household. She loves to play board games, spend time with family, laugh with friends, eat chips and salsa, and go on date nights.

ENDNOTES

1 Stomachs Icon Remake photo

2 Basal Metabolic Rate. http://en.wikipedia.org/wiki/Basal_metabolic_rate

3 FDA. http://www.fda.gov/downloads/Food/ResourcesForYou/Consumers/UCM079504.pdf. May 2007.

4 Institute of Medicine. Dietary Reference Intakes for Energy, Carbohydrate, Fiber, Fat, Fatty Acids, Cholesterol, Protein, and Amino Acids. Washington (DC): The National Academies Press; 2002. Page 15.

5 http://www.fda.gov/Food/IngredientsPackagingLabeling/LabelingNutrition/ucm079609.htm. Last Updated: 05/22/2016.

6 "Morality." *Merriam-Webster.com*. Merriam-Webster, n.d. Web. 29 Sept. 2014. <http://www.merriam-webster.com/dictionary/morality>.

7 November 3, 2003, https://www.barna.org/barna-update/article/5-barna-update/129-morality-continues-to-decay#.VCmDEVVdU4t www.barna.org written permission

8 "Detoxify." *Merriam-Webster.com*. Merriam-Webster, n.d. Web. 29 Sept. 2014. <http://www.merriam-webster.com/dictionary/detoxify>.

9 "Emotion." *Merriam-Webster.com*. Merriam-Webster, n.d. Web. 29 Sept. 2014. <http://www.merriam-webster.com/dictionary/emotion>.

10 "Jealousy." *Merriam-Webster.com*. Merriam-Webster, n.d. Web. 29 Sept. 2014. <http://www.merriam-webster.com/dictionary/jealousy>.

11 "Gossip." *Merriam-Webster.com*. Merriam-Webster, n.d. Web. 18 July 2016.

12 "Disciple." *Merriam-Webster.com*. Merriam-Webster, n.d. Web. 18 July 2016.

13 Jerajani, H. R. et al. "HEMATOHIDROSIS – A RARE CLINICAL PHENOMENON." *Indian Journal of Dermatology* 54.3 (2009): 290–292. *PMC*. Web. 28 Nov. 2016.

14 "Character." *Merriam-Webster.com*. Merriam-Webster, n.d. Web. 18 July 2016.

15 Mikel Burley (2012), Classical Samkhya and Yoga; An Indian Metaphysicsor Experience, Routledge, ISBN 978-0-415-64887-5.

16 James M. Nelson(209), Psychology, Religion, and Spirituality, Springer, ISBN 978-1-4419-2769-9, pages 78-82.

17 Barna Research Online, "Morality Continues to Decay," November 3, 2003. www.barna.org/cgi-bin/PagePressRelease.asp. Referenced with written permission. All rights reserved.

18 Colgan, Michael, Dr. "Blog Post; Maximum Movement, Optimum Strength," Web. <http://healthyreaders.com/category/dr-michael-colgan/>.

Made in the USA
Lexington, KY
07 June 2019